the blue book on health

edited by

Edward Vaizey

Politico's
PUBLISHING

First published in Great Britain 2002
by Politico's Publishing
8 Artillery Row
London SW1P 1RZ

A catalogue record for this book is available from the British Library.

ISBN 1 84275 043 7

Printed and bound by Creatve Print and Design
Designed and typeset by Politico's Design, design@politicos.co.uk

Contents

Acknowledgements

In July 2001 Michael Gove, Nicholas Boles and I decided to edit a book of essays on the future of the Conservative party. It seemed to us that the defeat the party had suffered at the polls in June 2001 meant that some urgent analysis was required about the reasons for that defeat and the way forward.

The result was the publication of *A Blue Tomorrow* in October 2001, a little over two months after we had had the idea. The speed of publication was down to the goodwill of all the many contributors and the support of Iain Dale at Politico's, who ensured a speedy and smooth editing and publication process.

A Blue Tomorrow has been a modest success. It has sold well and it has been widely discussed. It clearly filled a gap in the market – a desire by Conservative activists to read and absorb a wide range of challenging opinions about the party.

After publication, John Berry at Politico's suggested to me that I should edit and publish a series of books looking at different policy areas that the Conservatives would concentrate on. *The Blue Book on Health* is the result of his excellent advice. It is the first in what I hope will be a series of policy books on topics such as transport, education and crime, to be published at six monthly intervals. Once again, I am hugely indebted and grateful to the large numbers of contributors who have given their time and thoughts free of charge; to John Berry and Iain Dale for seeing through the logistics; and to Brooks Newmark and Richard Benyon for agreeing to underwrite the financial costs of the project. All contributors views are their own; all errors are mine.

The Blue Book on Health follows the spirit of *A Blue Tomorrow*. It is designed to give an overview of the debate on health policy from a wide range of perspectives, not necessarily all political and certainly not Conservative. It will, I hope, allow those with a passing interest in the subject to read in a little more depth about the issues being debated and discussed. It will also, I hope, help stimulate further debate in Conservative circles about the way ahead in this important policy area.

Edward Vaizey, March 2002

Notes on contributors

Edward Vaizey is the director of Consolidated Communications Public Affairs. He co-edited *A Blue Tomorrow* and writes and broadcasts regularly about the Conservative Party.

Mark Bassett is head of public policy at BUPA.

Andrew Cooper runs a market research company.

Stephen Evans is a member of Conservative Central Office's Policy Unit.

Dr Tim Evans (Ph.D) is Executive Director of Public Affairs at the Independent Healthcare Association.

Dr David Green (Ph.D) is Director of Civitas: the Institute for the Study of Civil Society (www.civitas.org.uk).

Johan Hjertqvist is manager of the Timbro Health Unit in Sweden.

Ruth Lea is head of the Policy Unit at the Institute of Directors.

Gerald Malone is a former Health Minister.

Michael McManus is a former parliamentary candidate and the author of a life of Jo Grimond.

Dr Kate Pickering is a GP and former parliamentary candidate.

Stephen Pollard is a senior fellow at the Centre for the New Europe, in Brussels, and at Civitas.

Dr Jonathan Reggler is co-ordinator of the Independent General Practitioners Association and member of the BMA General Practitioners committee.

Professor John Spiers (University of Glamorgan), an independent commentator on health care, is a former Chairman of The Patients Association. He is not a member of any political party.

Sean Williams is a member of the policy unit at Conservative Central Office.

Introduction

Edward Vaizey

Over the last six months, a fierce debate has been raging about the future of the National Health Service. For the first time for many years, the debate has not centred simply on the level of funding for this venerable institution, but more on whether it can survive in its present form.

One realises that the debate is serious when the *Observer*'s Health Editor, Anthony Browne, devotes a whole page in his paper to attacking the current system, concluding that:

> It is inevitable that a state monopoly offering free services will treat patients like mindless sheep, forcing them to accept whatever they are given . . . The Government can fiddle with [the NHS] as long as it likes, but the very structure of the NHS ensures it will never be world class.[1]

This situation presents a great opportunity for the Conservatives. Indeed, they have no option but to seize it. As Anatole Kaletsky pointed out, this debate may be the 'last best chance of political resurrection'[2] for the Conservatives. We have to engage in this debate, but the question we are faced with is how.

In the opening essay in this book, Andrew Cooper presents a trenchant analysis of what the Conservatives can and cannot get away with saying to the public. Just as he showed in *A Blue*

Tomorrow, unless we are fiercely honest with ourselves about how the public see the Conservative approach to the NHS, we will risk squandering our opportunity.

As Cooper points out, simply to mimic Labour's approach in opposition will not be enough. To say that everything was a disaster after Labour came to power is simply not credible. One of the main reasons that we lost power in 1997 was because the public did not trust us in key issues such as health and education. Similarly, scare stories based on the horror of individual patients' cases will not work for us, as it did not work for Kinnock.

What the public will appreciate is a more measured and thoughtful approach to the whole debate. To be fair to the Conservatives, many of the reforms put together in the 1990s would, if they had been left to bed down, probably have resulted in significant improvements in healthcare. Indeed, as the *Financial Times* pointed out in an editorial on Alan Milburn's key note policy speech made at the beginning of the year: 'the headline . . . might have read "The Tories were right all along" . . . Labour could have got there in 18 months if it had worked with what it inherited'.[3]

Milburn is slowly trying to modernise the NHS, but it remains the case that Labour seems to be committed to a centrally-funded system paid for by taxpayers. What is equally clear from this collection of essays is that there needs to be a radical reappraisal of how the NHS is funded and organised. In the 1990s, with GP fundholding and purchaser/provider splits, the Conservatives introduced a system that had market elements, allowing money to flow where it was most needed and for costs to become more transparent. The first term of the Labour

Government saw much of this good work undone. Now reform is on the agenda again.

One after another, almost all of the contributors to this book look at some sort of reinvention of the health service. What unties them is a number of beliefs. First, decision-making in health must be devolved down, if possible as far as the patient. Second, local solutions must be found, rather than central diktats from Whitehall. Finally, more private money must be brought into the system – simple increases in taxation will never ensure that enough money can be found.

Such recommendations are not set out to cut costs. Rather, they are put forward to turn the NHS from being a provider-focused organisation to a customer-centred one. As the Conservatives recognised in the 1990s, unless people are allowed to behave like customers, directing funds to where they are needed and being provided with a range of choices, the NHS will continue to be an inflexible monolith. That is why contributors such as Ruth Lea recommend an NHS passport, John Spiers a medical health account, Gerry Malone an endowment fund for individuals, Jonathan Reggler some form of charging, and David Green and Stephen Pollard a social insurance system and competing insurance providers. All these contributors, to an extent, sing in harmony. Give patients power and they will exercise it for the common good. More importantly, organisational reform such as this will ensure that we have an honest debate about what the NHS can provide. We need to have a core service that can be topped up, so that more private money can enter the system.

No system is perfect. As Stephen Pollard points out, the much lauded French system is economically unsustainable and relies on doctors being paid comparatively low wages. As Michael McManus also makes clear, we have had debates about decentralising and reforming the NHS almost since the day it was born, but radical change has never been achieved. And as Kate Pickering, a practising GP and former candidate shows, not all Conservatives want to move from a taxpayer funded system. There is no doubt at all that achieving radical change, or indeed advocating it, will be difficult. But change can be achieved, as Johan Hjertqvist shows in his essay on what is happening in Stockholm.

The Blue Book on Health is designed to be a primer. Many of the contributors are well-known in this field, and to experts their views will be familiar. It should be emphasised at this point that few are active Conservatives – and indeed almost all are politically neutral. I have asked the Conservative Policy Unit to contribute an overview of the state of the NHS as an appendix, as so many people ask for statistics. I must emphasise that its inclusion is not meant to brand any other contribution as "Conservative". Most are emphatically not, and can be picked up by any policy maker from any party. To the general reader interested in the debate on health, this is a chance to read considered views in depth and to gain some understanding on the nature and level of debate. I hope that it proves to be a useful companion as the debate continues.

Edward Vaizey, March 2002

1 The *Observer*, 7 October 2001

2 *The Times*, 29 November 2001

3 *Financial Times*, 16 January 2002

Trust in health

Why the Conservative Party must win back trust on the NHS, and how to start

Andrew Cooper

The NHS and Conservative decline

It is no coincidence that the decline and fall of the Conservative Party was accompanied by the steady emergence of a consensus that the National Health Service was in crisis. The future of both these formerly world-beating British institutions remains intertwined.

The common perception of Conservative attitudes to the NHS was a primary cause of the party's ignominious collapse to unelectability.[1] Changing that perception is a *sine qua non* of the party's political restoration – if it is to have one. This cannot be overstated. No single issue matters more. We were in power for a long period in which the NHS was not a very important political issue, and survived for a while longer in government having lost people's trust on the NHS. But it is another matter entirely to try and regain office from that position. If we are not trusted on the health service we will not win. It is as simple as that.

Rebuilding this trust is an urgent priority. The issue is ineluctably salient[2] and the Government is manifestly failing to live up to the expectations fuelled by its campaigning rhetoric.

But disappointment at Labour's failure will not liberate us. It will no doubt cause many people not to vote Labour. But most will not vote Conservative until, and unless, we have won back their trust. In the meantime, swelling disillusionment about Labour's failure to deliver improvements in the NHS will benefit the Liberal Democrats, not the Conservatives. Failure to address urgently the Conservative Party's fundamental NHS problem is likely, therefore, to prove not only a tactical mistake, but also a strategic disaster.

It is hard to conceive that we could win a general election while nearly two voters in five think, as they currently do, that 'the Conservative Party's attitude to public services is hostile'.[3] The point bears emphasis: nearly 40 per cent of the electorate think that our attitude towards the public services is characterised not merely by lack of concern, or even doctrinaire policy solutions, but by active hostility.

It should go without saying that our highest priority must be to understand, and respond to, this problem.

To start with we must understand how we got into this position – being honest, as we do so, about our own mistakes, and proportionate about those of the Labour government. But first we should understand clearly and learn lessons from Labour's handling of the NHS, both in opposition and, since 1997, in government.

A monster of Labour's making

It may well turn out to be the National Health Service that, in the end, breaks the Labour government.[4] The patience of the public is now exhausted.

It is a pleasing irony: the Labour Government has become as much a victim of its own rhetoric and branding as the Conservative Party before it.

In opposition the Labour Party lied riotously about public spending on health, and gloried in every scrap of evidence that the NHS was failing. Labour deliberately created the myth of a Tory government that was viciously cutting health funding and trying to privatise the NHS by stealth, and used the Tory gargoyle they had thus designed as the counterpoint to Labour's agenda for change, and their all-embracing chorus that 'things can only get better'.

Long before Tony Blair's ludicrous (and, from his point of view, unfortunately memorable) hyperbole, on the eve of the 1997 election, that there were '24 hours to save the NHS', most voters had been persuaded that the increasingly obvious problems in the National Health Service were linked to the apparent fact that the Tories didn't use it, didn't believe in it, and didn't care about it. From these assumptions it was a small logical leap to accept Labour's claims that the Tories were, therefore, cutting spending on the NHS in order to fund tax cuts for the few, and that the Conservative agenda was one of creeping privatisation.

Most voters were optimistic about the prospects for the NHS once Labour came to power. It was entirely consistent with Labour's brand that they both cared deeply about the National Health Service and would actually spend more money on it, rather than merely pretend to, as people thought the Major government had done. So, it was reasonable to assume that improvements would quickly follow.

If – as Labour has asserted, and most people believed – the obvious problems in the NHS were caused by under-funding and lack of political commitment, Labour was plainly the antidote to both. Yet nothing happened. Improvements did not follow. If anything, casual empiricism and the tenor of media coverage suggested that in many parts of the country NHS services were getting worse, not better.

In the absence of any actual improvements to brag about (indeed, in the face of lengthening waiting lists and periodic health crises) Tony Blair began to treat public spending as a proxy for delivery – almost as a measure of output rather than input.

By the summer of 1998, the Prime Minister had elevated higher spending to be the *raison d'être* of his government, telling William Hague:

> He and his party have still not worked out why they lost the last election. They lost it because people want additional expenditure on schools and hospitals. They now know that we will provide that money for schools and hospitals, whereas the Conservative Party would take it away.[5]

Towards the end of Tony Blair's first term the failure of increased spending to yield improved services became an increasing complaint among voters. The question most people were asking about public spending was no longer 'where's the money coming from?' but 'where's the money going?'

By the time of the general election, most voters were intensely disappointed with Labour's record – on the NHS above all else. But qualitative research revealed, decisively, that most people also felt that at least Labour meant well; their heart was in the right place; they were trying. The Tories, on the other hand, showed no signs at all of accepting their share of the blame for the problems of the NHS. They talked as if all the troubles of the health service began on 1 May 1997,[6] and didn't seem that interested in the subject anyway – going through the motions of talking about it from time to time because the rules of engagement demanded it, rather than because they truly cared.

Frustration at the Government's failure to live up to its promises on the NHS was undoubtedly one of the main reasons why many people who had voted Labour in 1997 were unwilling to do so in 2001. But hardly any of these people felt able to vote Conservative; rather more switched to the Liberal Democrats, and more still simply didn't vote at all. This pattern can be seen clearly when opinion polls ask voters which party has the best policies on the NHS: Labour's rating has fallen by more than a quarter over the past few years, but virtually none of those losing faith in Labour policies have turned to the Conservative Party.[7]

There was surprisingly little enthusiasm for Labour at the 2001 election. It was a landslide grudgingly bestowed. Liam Fox, Conservative Party Health Spokesman since the mid-point in the last Parliament, was right to point out to the Party's 2001 annual conference that Labour merely 'got the benefit of the doubt'. He was wrong to go on flatly to assert that 'they won't get it next time'.[8] It is dangerous, and unfounded, complacency.

Unless the Conservative Party comes to terms with the truth of how voters view the party and its attitude towards the health service, and unless it responds wholeheartedly, it is all too possible that Labour will be given the benefit of the doubt at the next election too – because, quite simply, the doubt is about us and whether we can be trusted.

Losing trust

We must start by being completely honest and explicit about the reasons behind the loss of trust in Conservative motives towards the NHS. This does not necessarily mean that past Conservative governments were wrong to do the things they did. That is not the point. But the consequence – in many cases unseeable or irrelevant at the time – of things that the Conservative Party said and did during its long period of government during the 1980s and 1990s was to build a picture of a party that did not seem really to understand, care about, or wish to preserve, the National Health Service:

- Conservative governments had other priorities – fundamentally economic ones, and for a decade, at least, took relatively little interest in the NHS. The net effect was the impression of a party whose primary concern about the health service was to control its cost;
- Conservative leaders were unembarrassed about proclaiming that they did not themselves use the NHS and for many voters this equated to a lack of personal commitment, and hence a lack of political commitment;

- Conservative governments presided over, or at least coincided with (voters are unlikely ever to make a distinction between the two) the emergence of serious and apparently chronic problems of capacity in the NHS;
- The Conservative Party championed and introduced reforms, to the NHS – in particular the introduction of a purchaser/provider split – which were condemned by much of the medical profession for 'commercialising' the NHS – reinforcing our image as being more interested in applying 'market solutions' to the NHS than in delivering quality services to patients;
- Conservative governments also backed the rationalisation of hospital services whose effect was to shut down numerous small local hospitals in favour of fewer, larger, better-equipped, ones. This policy created innumerable pockets of bitter opposition to the Conservative approach – which many felt were motivated by the search for cost savings, not the desire to deliver better services. The policy also resulted in an actual reduction in the number of hospital beds – apparently tangible (though misleading) 'proof' of Tory cuts;
- The overall image of the Conservative Party was inconsistent with the thought that we 'cared' about public services, and about those who have to rely on the NHS.

These perceptions were extremely significant in the collapse in the fortunes of the Conservative Party. They have changed very little during the five years that the party has so far been in opposition. During the last Parliament there was insufficient recognition that until these negatives are addressed our message will simply not get through, and as a result little real effort was made to overcome them.

Ironically, the Conservative Party did identify the shift in public mood during the Parliament. It recognised that people were beginning to ask where the money was going and spent millions on billboard advertising that said 'You've paid the tax, so where are the operations?'[9]

The Party's problem was that, although it had identified the public mood on public services, its ability to campaign credibly on Labour's failure to deliver was severely limited by the fact that virtually nothing had been done since 1997 to address the fundamental distrust that voters have for the Party's approach to the NHS. Furthermore, no critique of Labour's record on health, however resonant, would get a really positive reaction from voters unless it was accompanied by a clear and credible positive proposition – which the Conservative campaign, despite four years in which to think about it, was never in a position to offer.

As a result the party all but abandoned the NHS as a campaigning issue during the general election – an extraordinary tactical decision given the paramount importance of the health service to most voters, and the government's growing vulnerability on the issue.[10]

William Hague, and his advisers, should have taken seriously from the outset the vital importance of rebuilding trust in Conservative instincts towards public services. Having failed to do that they should at least have understood that general election campaigns – when voters pay more attention to politics than at any other time – are the best chance we get to present a picture of what the party stands for, its values and character.

In 1997 Conservatives were judged, as the venerable commentator Anthony Howard has put it, to be 'a loathsome, odious party'. Five years on, he adds, 'they are faced by a firm mindset on the part of the public which sees their party not just as useless, but repugnant as well'.[11]

The Conservatives' 2000 general election campaign should have been a determined effort to challenge these vile impressions of Tories. The campaign's remarkably perverse accomplishment was to achieve the opposite – compounding rather than challenging bitterly negative perceptions, which had in any case been exacerbated in two further respects during the last Parliament:

- We behave like politicians, and – compounded by Labour's broken promises, and their lack of humility in response to those broken promises – trust in politicians is at an all time low. The general motives of politicians are held in contempt, and most voters think that politicians habitually evade the truth, and prefer silly Westminster games to serious consideration of ways to deal with Britain's real problems – like the state of the NHS;
- People think we treat the NHS as a political football. The reason that they think this is that all too often it is true. We have too often been guilty of political and intellectual inconsistency, of jumping on any bandwagon generated by the media however fatuous – and of putting our arguments with intemperate language and with no sense of self-awareness.

It is no wonder therefore that when Conservatives appear on

radio or television speaking about how bad things are in the NHS most people have two reactions:

a) That most of the problems have their root in Tory policies (and so our point is hypocritical – and also annoying because we apparently think people are too stupid to notice that we are being hypocritical), and;
b) That our motive for talking down the NHS is that we want to privatise it (because that is always the Conservative 'big idea' for things in the public sector) – and 'look what privatisation did to the railways'.

The Conservative Party does not, in marketing parlance, have permission currently to talk about how bad things are in the health service, just as we do not have permission to criticise Labour's management of the NHS without acknowledging our own past mistakes. We also have no business impugning Labour's motives. Even the most disgruntled consumers of the NHS accept that the Labour government 'means well' – it is one of the factors that makes their failure to deliver improvements all the more puzzling and frustrating.

How to be heard again

The American political theorist James Stimson[12] has developed an interesting thesis that public opinion does not, as psephologists have tended to assume, exist in a stable state characterised by occasional discontinuities and abrupt changes of direction, but by a process of systemic continuous change.

Stimson describes a world in which individuals constantly

adjust to, and sub-consciously re-evaluate, the impact of public policies. Party competition theory – the orthodoxy of political scientists – asserts that party politics is a competitive game of incremental policy change to keep in step with what the public wants. Political parties, Stimson concludes, must operate within a 'zone of acquiescence' – the spatial representation of the public's policy preferences, which will often be vague, and at times contradictory.

If public opinion is not stable, however, but continuously evolving relative to the actions of the policy makers – with voters responding to changing situations, and to their experience and perception of the impact of policy – political parties can and will find themselves carried outside the zone of acquiescence. That is what happened to the Conservative Party.

In the late 1970s and 1980s voters wanted a robust government to turn Britain around, neuter the unions, restore equilibrium to the economy, and reduce the reach, and the cost, of the state. By the late 1980s and early 1990s people increasingly began to see the public services as a high priority, and to feel that the characteristics they had liked in Conservative governments did not suit the new agenda.

Underlying Stimson's theory is the human observation that the demands and expectations of voters will at times be neither reasonable nor rational. People are readily capable of believing – and wanting – contradictory things, often simultaneously. And, of course, the grass is almost always greener on the other side.

But the turning circle of a government is considerably larger than that of individual voters. Politicians continue on a course whose co-ordinates were based on a clear set of public preferences. But when those preferences change – swinging into reverse – parties end up overshooting the zone of acquiescence.

This is what has happened to the Conservative Party. It cannot postpone any longer the moment when it honestly faces, and openly debates, the fact that most voters continue to regard us as a malign irrelevance. We must accept, finally, that this is our central problem and that until it is resolved we will play little or no meaningful part in the great political debates of our age.

Until we re-enter the zone of acquiescence, not even the most ingenious policy for the NHS will overcome entrenched negative public perceptions about our motives. None of our Conservative ideas to improve the National Health Service will be heard with open minds, and none of our arguments believed, until we have with discipline and urgency started to eliminate our long-standing negatives.[13]

Restoring trust

We do not have to look far for our starting point. Conservatives should remember the wisdom that won back the people's trust the last time we were in opposition. The 1979 Conservative Party general election manifesto concluded:

> We make no lavish promises. The repeated disappointment of rising expectations has led to a marked loss of faith in politicians' promises. . . . Most people, in their hearts, know that Britain has to come to terms with

> reality. They no longer have any time for politicians who try to gloss over the harsh facts of life. Most people want to be told the truth, and to be given a clear lead towards the action needed for recovery. The years of make-believe and false optimism are over. It is time for a new beginning.

If we are to win back trust in Conservative instincts towards the National Health Service, our narrative on the NHS must begin with an admission of where and how we went wrong. If, as it often seems to do, our proposition integrally requires voters to accept that in 1997 they wrongly judged the state of the NHS, and the effect of Tory government's policies, then we may as well give up now.[14]

Public perceptions have deep roots. It is twenty years since Margaret Thatcher felt it necessary to proclaim at the Conservative Party conference that 'the NHS is safe with us'. It is fifteen years since that the *British Medical Journal*, with characteristic pomposity, declared the National Health Service to be in terminal decline and the presidents of the three royal medical colleges – the great and good of the medical world – called on Mrs Thatcher's Government to 'save our health service'.[15] It was a full decade later before the Conservative Party was finally ejected from office – ten years during which the caricature of our attitudes towards the NHS festered menacingly.

Until we are ready at last to concede this point, to deal with it, and to move on, we will remain stuck with the hoary negatives that led to two successive crushing electoral defeats; until then, our arguments about the NHS will continue to fall on deaf ears.[16]

Being proportionate: crisis, what crisis?

Acknowledging the past, however, is not enough. As well as being honest and straightforward about ourselves, we must be equally clear and truthful about the scale, and nature, of the problems in the NHS.

Almost everyone has – or knows someone who has – experience of an NHS failure. And virtually everybody expresses their feelings about the health service through personal anecdote. Two thirds of the public think that the NHS is in 'poor shape' and three times as many people think it is getting worse as think it is getting better (though nearly half believe it is 'staying about the same'). But, at the same time, 86 per cent of people say they are happy with the care they get from their GP, and 77 per cent are happy with the hospital treatment they have received.[17] Furthermore, 91 per cent are satisfied with the way that doctors do their job and 94 per cent with how nurses do their job.[18]

So although there is a common *perception* that the NHS is in crisis, there is also a common *experience* that it is still performing satisfactorily, and an almost universal view that doctors and nurses are doing their jobs well. As Professor Anthony King has noted, although the actual number of people who have a bad experience of the NHS is relatively low, 'As dissatisfied patients and their families talk not only to each other, but also to friends, neighbours and chance acquaintances, the number of people in Britain who have recently been regaled with NHS complaints and horror stories must number in the tens of millions'.[19] This reality is vastly compounded by the media, which hysterically overlooks the reality that there are tens of thousands of successful interactions with the NHS for each one that goes seriously wrong.[20] Each individual instance of poor treatment, or worse, by the NHS brings distress – or sometimes tragedy – to a family somewhere, and affects a much larger community of interest. But, as the party of the Dangerous Dogs Act ought to remember, hard cases make bad policy.

We must not, of course, miss the point that nearly one patient in five is not happy with the standard of hospital care they received, and more than one in eight are dissatisfied with some aspect of the service provided by their GP.[21] That is unacceptable. The NHS is not as good as it could or should be. But we must be proportionate. Actual experiences of the NHS – an abiding and overwhelming majority who are satisfied with the service they have had – suggest that the NHS is definitely not on the brink of fundamental breakdown. People overwhelmingly object to the length of time that the NHS makes them wait. Waiting times are in some cases scandalously long. But the great majority of people also believe that when they are treated, they are treated well. More than 80 per cent think that waiting times for operations and for treatment in A&E units are 'often far too long'. But 80 per cent also believe that 'if you are really ill, the NHS looks after you'.[22]

In 1998, 91 per cent of voters said they were satisfied with the treatment provided by the health service overall. By January 2002 that figure had fallen to 83 per cent.[23] The fact that 8 per cent of the population have become dissatisfied with the NHS during the last four years puts the scale of the problem in the right perspective – it is a significant slippage. But, objectively, the satisfaction rate for the NHS as a whole is still remarkably high.

The same narrative is reflected in data collected by the British Social Attitudes Survey.[24] This shows a very slight reduction in satisfaction with every aspect of the NHS that involves waiting – whether for outpatient appointments, non-emergency operations, appointments to see consultants, or trying to see a Doctor in an Accident and Emergency Department. Waiting lists are plainly a focal point of considerable general disgruntlement. There is a level of queuing that people are prepared to accept as the price of having a National Health Service that is free at the point of use, but over the last few years, waiting lists have gone beyond that level.[25] This frustration was fuelled by the fact that waiting *times*, which fell markedly between 1987 and 1996, rose during the second half of the last decade – though still less than half their level in the mid 1980s.[26]

But the British Social Attitudes Survey also finds that in other respects the NHS is perceived to be improving slightly, not getting worse. There is, for example, increased satisfaction with the general condition of hospital buildings, while satisfaction with the quality of medical treatment delivered by GPs and hospitals is at the same level as it was five years ago, and higher than a decade ago.

Conservatives should, therefore, proceed with caution, and not overstate the extent of crisis, or the readiness of the British people to countenance very radical plans for reform – especially when those come from a Conservative Party whose motives are not yet trusted.

It is never an edifying sight to see politicians trying their hardest to make a problem seem worse than it is. For politicians who expect some day to serve in government it is a tactical boomerang – as Labour has discovered.

There is a further tactical case for being proportionate in our rhetoric about the NHS. It is facile to suppose that the vast sums of taxpayers' money that have been pumped into the National Health Service since 1999 will yield no improvements at all. However crude the investment strategy, and whatever the level of waste, those Conservatives who prophesy doom for the NHS run the risk of being proved wrong, as well as the likelihood of seeming mean spirited.[27]

It is especially important for the Conservative Party to heed this fact, not because we are on the brink of office, but because we are so far from it. Voters are cynical. They are also increasingly sophisticated in their reading of the media. Every political pronouncement that they hear (and most people screen out most political statements) is subjected to the test of motive.

We should at all times try to be honest, proportionate, decent and likable. It shouldn't need to be pointed out – but does – that people are more likely to hear, absorb and accept an argument that is put in such a way. It is a principle put magnificently into practice by Shadow Home Secretary Oliver Letwin. He has understood that noting Labour's good intentions strengthens the impact of any subsequent criticism of them and makes it much more difficult for Ministers to evade questions by Parliamentary bluster – as well as making us seem more reasonable and less nasty.[28]

When we address ourselves to the National Health Service, we should be trying to communicate that though we made mistakes in the past, and accept responsibility for those mistakes, we care about the NHS, are committed to it, and are working hard on policies to improve the NHS. We should be positive as well as honest. That should always be our practice.

If a party that is suspected of malign motives towards the National Health Service wishes to persuade people that its intentions are, in fact, benign, it should not talk about how badly the NHS is doing, and how great are its problems, but how well the NHS is doing and how important it is to build on what is good and deal constructively with what is not.

The depth of negative perceptions about Conservative attitudes to the NHS, and our responsibility for its problems, imposes an inverse logic to our strategy. The more we point out how bad things are under Labour, the more that people's real disaffection with Labour is mitigated by irritation at how little we 'get it', and by the impression that we are talking down the NHS because we hold some desire to undermine or privatise it.

It is integral to this approach that we also recognise – especially given the present hostility towards politicians and their yah-boo habits – that few negative points will hit home unless they are accompanied by a positive proposal. Without it people tend to regard criticism as pointless carping. Unless we explicitly draw attention to our alternative to the government's approach, many people will default to the instinct that if we were in government we would be doing the same things as Labour (and if they were in opposition they would be making the same jibes as we are doing) – a common reaction to the things we say on many topics, and one that frequently emasculates the impact of our response to events.

The more we couch our awareness of much-needed improvements in the context of strong positive, even optimistic, comment about the foundations of the NHS, the greater the leverage we gain, and the less likely people are to keep on giving Labour the benefit of the doubt.

The realities of public attitudes, and the entrenched perceptions of our values and motives, carry clear lessons for Conservatives as we think and talk about the future of the National Health Service. They draw us towards certain policy conclusions or directions of policy – and away from others – and suggest some straightforward disciplines about how we explain our point of view.

The public spending cul-de-sac

The public finds the whole subject of public spending bewildering. For a start, most people are predisposed to disbelieve any and every statistic that they ever hear leave the mouth of a politician and it is hard, if not impossible, to talk for long about public spending without disappearing into a morass of statistics that, even if heard and comprehended, will not be believed.

Furthermore, we know that statistics about public spending won't be believed because the numbers involved are so large as to be simply beyond comprehension. Most people don't understand the difference between billions and millions, and many people use the two terms almost interchangeably.[29]

These are good enough reasons for any politician to avoid talking in detail about the level of public spending. For Conservatives there is another fundamental reason: until we have changed the underlying perception of our character almost nobody believes what we say on the subject. It simply defies the common view of the core branding of both main parties to conceive that the Conservative Party would spend more on public services than Labour.

We will not win an argument that we would be more generous than Labour in funding the NHS (and many Conservatives would regard it as an odd argument to wish to win), so we should not start one. There is a strong case for honouring Labour's spending commitments – giving us time to put in place constructive reforms. There is no case for trying to undermine or outstrip them.

The privatisation trap

Conservatives must also be wary of policy initiatives that are capable of being interpreted as privatisation – which would serve only to reinforce our negative stereotypes.

Proposals whose objective is to encourage private health

insurance, or increase the level of private sector management and financial involvement in the NHS, will make our position worse, not better. We have to establish in the public mind that our intentions are constructive, and our values benign, before we can hope to persuade voters that the future of the NHS will need to involve much more partnership activity with the private sector.

A transparency agenda

Instead of getting stuck in a stalemate over the level of public spending, or drawn into reinforcing our caricature as a party obsessed with the privatisation of public services, we should respond to the huge clamour for transparency and honesty about the NHS. Doing so will help to move the debate about the NHS, and about healthcare more broadly, in a constructive Conservative direction.

It is a very common cry from voters that they don't know 'where all the money goes'. Conservatives should respond.

At the last two general elections, the Conservative Party has advocated giving voters an annual statement of how their taxes are spent. The party has always undervalued this policy. It is a small and simple step, but one which would be enormously welcome.

As the debate about the NHS rages on, and the proportion of our national income spent on the health service rises, we should consider a more detailed level of transparency: not only telling people how much of their money has gone to the NHS, but also how the NHS spent it – under broad headings of activity.

Underpinning this should be a process of scrutiny on an unprecedented scale. Conservatives should be the champions of what Nick Gibb MP has termed a 'cheque-stub audit'. Most people have an unshakeable conviction that a lot of the tax they pay towards the NHS is wasted, and never gets through to services. They are, no doubt, correct and Conservative spokesmen have often made the same argument in criticising Labour's record.

But we have never made a substantial positive response to the point. The Conservative Party should take the lead in poring over NHS budgets, providing detailed answers to the question where does the money go, and, in the process, identifying actual waste, and red tape that would, at last, enable us to give convincing detail to our popular and frequent, but rarely substantiated, assertion that a Conservative government would ensure that taxpayers' money was spent more efficiently. We would be able to be explicit and precise in attacking the waste and bureaucracy that so angers voters – advancing a fundamental Conservative principle.

No, you haven't paid your stamp

Transparency about the NHS also obligates us to think seriously about the national insurance system. We must put an end to the great lie about national insurance contributions – which every government since World War II has allowed to persist. This is not just a point of rationalist purity. Being honest about national insurance will create a much greater level of understanding about the pressures on the NHS, and help create a climate in which constructive Conservative ideas, put in a civilised way, will be heard and believed.

It is an overwhelmingly common misconception that the national insurance system means that each working adult has, in effect, paid in advance for the healthcare they need. 'I've paid my stamp' is one of the most frequent refrains in focus group discussions about the NHS. Most people think that their national insurance contributions go into a discrete fund, earmarked for them – the Beveridge equivalent of saving for a rainy day. This total misapprehension has been encouraged, or at least overlooked, by successive governments because it is a fiction that helps to disguise the real level of taxation needed to fund current spending. Funding the year-on-year activities of central government consumes all of the money that most people have assumed was being put aside to pay for their health and welfare needs later in life; the 10 per cent or so of their income that most people pay in national insurance is not 'a stamp', it is, simply, tax.

The national insurance lie has a pervasive effect on attitudes to NHS provision because it underlies most people's instinctive resistance to incremental charging within the National Health Service, and is one of the reasons why many people rule out any kind of private medical insurance. If you believe you have already paid for the treatment you need in the NHS – over the years through national insurance – why on earth should you be expected to pay more, or to pay someone else to provide the service instead?

If, in these and other ways, Conservatives embrace the principles of transparency and honesty we will not only gain re-admission to the political mainstream, but also liberate constructive Conservative Party thinking on the NHS, increasing the prospect that both will, in the future, thrive.

---

1 At the last election 37 per cent of voters gave as their main reason for being reluctant to vote Conservative the perception that 'they wouldn't improve services like the NHS' (ICM call-back poll for the BBC, June 2001). A YouGov poll for the *Daily Telegraph* found in October 2001 that 52 per cent think that 'The Conservatives are not really interested in public services like the NHS and education'.

2 In recent years only the war against terrorism – fleetingly in the weeks following 11 September 2001 – has come above the NHS in MORI's ranking of the 'most important issues facing Britain'. The proportion of voters regarding the NHS as the most, or second-most, important issue facing Britain rose, according to MORI data, from 11 per cent in 1984 to 27 per cent in 1990, 29 per cent in 1993, 37 per cent in 1996, 39 per cent in 1999, and 48 per cent in 2001. In January February 2002, the equivalent figure was 72 per cent.

3 An ICM poll in January 2002 found that 37 per cent of voters agreed with this statement, more than 45 per cent of those voters expressing a view one way or the other.

4 A YouGov poll for the *Daily Telegraph* in January 2002 found that only 26 per cent thought the government was performing well on the NHS (only 1 per cent saying 'very well'), while 72 per cent felt they were performing badly (36 per cent saying 'very badly').

5 Tony Blair, 22 July 1998, Hansard col.1116

6 When it is put to Shadow Health Secretary Liam Fox that the Conservative often speaks as if the problems in the NHS began on 1 May 1997, he responds (e.g. interview during BBC 'NHS Day', 18 February 2002) by asserting that under-funding in the NHS dates back to 1963. This is a point only made in order to avoid directly having to accept Conservative responsibility for some of the problems in the NHS. Since the widespread experience of failings in the NHS was such a major reason why so many people wouldn't vote Conservative in 1997 it seems futile to be coy about the fact. We

are much more likely to persuade people to take our current views on the NHS seriously if we acknowledge that we made mistakes in the past, and that the NHS was already failing when Labour came to office. Denying things that everyone else regards as obvious truths just reminds voters of why they were glad to get rid of us.

7 ICM data shows that, when asked to choose which of the two main parties had the best policies for the NHS, Labour's rating fell from 56 per cent to 40 per cent between June 1999 and June 2001. Over the same period the number thinking the Conservative Party had the best policies rose by just 1 per cent, from 19 per cent to 20 per cent. The rest of those disaffected with Labour's approach opted for either 'neither party' or 'don't know'. In February 2002, MORI found that of the 72 per cent who think the NHS is among the most important issues, 40 per cent believe Labour has the best policy, and only 15 per cent favour Conservative policies.

8 Liam Fox, speech to the Conservative Party Conference, Blackpool, 9 October 2001.

9 This advertising campaign, devised by the Conservative Party's Director of Research Rick Nye in association with the party's advertising agency Yellow M, ran in January 2001. Most academic and journalistic accounts of the 2001 election campaign agree that it was the line of attack with which Labour were most uncomfortable, and Labour strategists were both amazed and delighted when the Conservative Party ceased to use it.

10 The conviction that the Conservative Party should simply ignore crucial issues and concentrate on less salient ones lay at the heart of the 'core vote strategy' and ensured that those voters who had felt unable to vote for us in 1997 had little reason to feel differently in 2001 and the sad but predictable consequence was a second defeat that was a virtual photocopy of the first.

11 Anthony Howard, *The Times*, 26 February 2002

12 Professor of Political Science, University of North Carolina – his intriguing theory of systemic cycles of public opinion is described in his book *Public Opinion in America – moods, cycles and swings* (Westview Press, 1991), and summarised, where I encountered it, in 'Apathetic Landslide', Pippa Norris's fascinating analysis of the 2001 general election result in *Britain Votes 2001* (Oxford University Press).

13 The crudeness and pervasiveness of the Conservative Party's image-problem can be gauged from the fact that, even in 2002 – five years after leaving office – qualitative research asking floating voters what the two main parties mean when they speak of 'change' in the NHS concludes that Labour means 'increasing nurses' pay', and Conservatives mean 'privatisation'.

14 As an illustration of the scale of the problem, an ICM poll in January 2000 found that 56 per cent of those expressing a view thought that Margaret Thatcher was most to blame for the crisis in the NHS, compared with 22 per cent who blamed Tony Blair most, and only 4 per cent who named Alan Milburn.

15 Mrs Thatcher's response was to commission the *Griffiths Report*, which was to herald many of the changes that the same medical professionals were later to execrate.

16 It is ironic that a recurring Conservative criticism of Tony Blair and his government

is that they refuse to accept responsibility for their policy mistakes, and try endlessly to spin their way away from the truth, yet many Conservatives are guilty of exactly the same behaviour, hence the fact that voters now regard it as the standard for all politicians.

17 Gallup poll, published in the *Daily Telegraph*, 14 January 2002.

18 MORI poll conducted for the British Medical Association, 7–13 February 2002.

19 'Ailing NHS in desperate need of a cure', *Daily Telegraph*, 14 January 2002

20 It was striking that Tony Blair, in his BBC TV interview with Nicky Campbell on 'NHS Day', 18 February 2002, directly confronted *Daily Mail* columnist Ann Leslie about that newspaper's predilection for doom-laden front-page stories about individual cases of bad treatment in hospitals.

21 18 per cent of people are dissatisfied with some aspect the treatment they have received in hospital, 12 per cent with some aspect of their treatment by a GP, according to Gallup, op. cit.

22 Data from Gallup, op. cit.

23 Ibid.

24 Data from the British Social Attitudes Survey contained in *Social Trends 31* section 8.8 (Office for National Statistics, 2001)

25 The number of people waiting for in-patient admission ranged between about 450,000 and about 750,000 in the period between the foundation of the NHS and the late 1980s. The total broke through the one million barrier in the early 1990s, peaking at nearly 1.3 million in the late 1990s. It now stands at about 1.1 million – nearly 2 per cent of the population.

26 Figures from the report of the House of Commons Select Committee, 1999, Table 4.15.3.

27 Public expenditure on the NHS will increase by 27 per cent in real terms in the five years between 1999/00 and 2003/04.

28 For example, Oliver Letwin's reply to a statement on nationality, immigration and asylum, 7 February 2002 (*Hansard* column 1029) began: 'Some months ago, when the Home Secretary first made a statement about his proposals for changing the UK's asylum arrangements, I responded that the aim of the Conservative party—like that of the Government—is to see the establishment of an asylum system that is humane, effective and fair; that rapidly provides a safe home for the innocent victims of persecution; and that, at the same time, prevents the asylum system being misused as a means of evading our immigration rules. I have since reiterated that position, and I restate it today. We welcome unreservedly the fact that the Home Secretary is genuinely trying to make those joint aims a reality.'

29 In focus group discussions about the NHS, almost invariably someone will make the point that the money spent on the Millennium Dome could have 'sorted out the problems of the health service'. The £768 million in question represents about one seventieth of the annual NHS budget. Similarly, when the last Conservative govern-

ment was proposing to replace the Royal Yacht, the common reason for opposing the idea was that the £60 million involved could 'go a long way in the NHS' – when, at the time, it would have kept the NHS running for slightly less than four hours.

The NHS – not bust, just the wrong paymaster

Gerald Malone

The purpose of this essay is not to crow over the corpse of the NHS, now understood by patients and doctors, but not yet politicians, to have reached the end of its useful life, but to focus the debate about healthcare provision on a neglected problem that lies at the heart of both the UK and US healthcare systems – the fact that, in both, patients rely on someone else to pay for their healthcare, a phenomenon known technically as 'third party payments'. In the UK patients rely on the taxpayer to fund their care. In the US insurers and health management organisations pick up the tab for the majority, Medicare and Medicaid schemes sort out the rest.

Labour's traditional knee jerk objection to the US health system, and much of UK non-NHS care, is that it is mostly private. For the patient that is not the case. From his point of view, as in the UK, healthcare is seen as a 'right' for which someone else will eventually pick up the tab. Whether it is an employer, or even an individual paying healthcare premiums, or the taxpayer who foots the bill, is irrelevant. Rarely in either country is the patient the paymaster.

What drives the dynamics of health care spending in both the US and the UK is that, from the consumer's point of view consumption of healthcare is cost free – 'free at the point of delivery' is the UK all-party politicians' mantra. It is a remarkable phenomenon that, alone of any other service widely used by the public in any developed country, health care systems are supermarkets without checkouts or barriers to entry. Little wonder that even exponential rises in spending fail to meet insatiable demand.

Reductio ad absurdum, the point becomes obvious: if government were today to take leave of its senses and initiate a policy of paying 100 per cent of the cost of new cars, most motorists would rush to the Jaguar showroom, passing previously acceptable Ford Mondeos on the forecourt. Manufacturers, sensing that price resistance in motorists was a thing of the past, would gold plate products, encourage regular replacement and use the latest technologies since the cost to drivers would be nil. That is the model that is the NHS, free at the point of delivery, free from cost constraint from the patient's perspective, a target for producers who use self-serving PR to whip up patient demand for the latest 'wonder remedy'. It is hardly surprising that inflation in health care costs is the highest of any economic sector.

Stop asking the wrong questions

Since the NHS was established in 1948, healthcare has replaced Anglicanism as the national religion. As the monarch is Defender of the Faith, so successive Health Secretaries have been cast as Defenders of the NHS. Getting more cash from the Treasury has been their main goal and test of their political virility, not improving health. National debate long ago descended to Punch and Judy levels of irrelevancy. The testosterone, or in one case oestrogen, levels of Health Secretaries have been measured by a yardstick that is irrelevant to any proper assessment of healthcare provision – the 'How much?' question.

In the UK we spend about 7 per cent of GDP on health care. Other European countries spend around 9 per cent, the US 14 per cent. We are 'bad'. They are 'good'. The Prime Minister has casually committed the government to match European levels of spending. Why? Spending is not virtuous if it brings with it no measurable improvements to healthcare services, or outcomes. Record increases on NHS spending over the last 30 years have brought nothing but misery for patients, doctors and politicians alike. There has never been a moment when the British Medical Association has not claimed that 'morale is at an all time low'. Why they all defend this system which in their own terms is failing badly is a mystery.

Does healthcare work?

In 1994, during a round of introductory ministerial briefing, the writer asked bemused officials in the Department of Health how much of the then £32 billion budget 'worked' – i.e. was proven to make people better. Even Railtrack can tell you how many trains run on time. It took ten days to come up with an answer – a mind bogglingly low 10 per cent. In the frosty discussion that followed the reason for this pitiful result rapidly emerged. Patients had no interest in whether healthcare brought benefits. Their priority was to receive rapid treatment for real or imagined conditions. Apart from obvious cases of self evidently successful treatment, like emergency or elective surgery, there was little focus on measurements to prove that complex procedures whose outcomes were difficult to evaluate did any good. Hospital readmission rates were the standard measure of quality, but that only measured what had gone badly wrong, not whether a procedure had been beneficial in the first place.

In the few areas where pioneering academics had carefully studied the outcomes of certain common procedures, they were found to have been pointless. Fitting grommets to children's ears is probably the best-known example. On close scrutiny, a procedure that had been commonplace across the NHS was judged pointless. The dynamics of a third party payment healthcare system do not encourage probing of that sort. It is uncomfortable for incumbent practitioners and patients have no economic interest in asking. If it's not their cash that's on the line trusting the doctor is the line of least resistance.

The most startling example of this disinterest in the 'does it work?' question is in the provision of prescription medicines. For a General Practitioner treatment ends at the point when a patient is handed a prescription and leaves the surgery. Does he bother to take it to the chemist? If he does, does he take it according to instructions – critical in the case of drugs like antibiotics? If these things happen, is the patient cured? No-one knows and £13 billion worth of drugs per annum, rising at the annual rate of 10 per cent, is stuffed down throats or dangerously clogs up the nations bathroom cabinets.

It's good, not bad, healthcare that is a growth sector

In a time of recession, when consumer spending is hailed as the saviour of the economy, why is it that healthcare spending is consciously capped? No one worries about the percentage of GDP spent on cars, food, shoes or travel. When did you last hear a politician call for spending on housing to be brought up to European levels? It is a 'good thing' for the economy if spending in these sectors is buoyant.

A nationally provided healthcare system has an interest in containing expenditure, simply to keep public spending totals under control. If the sales manager burst through Henry Ford's office at his Detroit HQ shouting 'demand for cars is shooting through the roof', it would be champagne all round and a trip to Wall Street to raise the capital needed for increased production. In the NHS the Soviet style command economy of failed demand management provokes only gloom when demand rises and another assault on the No.11 cash citadel beckons.

If healthcare is to play its proper role as a highly skilled service industry in a growing economy it needs free access to capital to meet the demands of paying customers.

He who pays the Piper . . .

Re-establishing the patient as the purchaser as well as the consumer of health care is essential if the sector is to become capable of attracting the capital needed to fund care that patients want and are prepared to pay for, as well as cut out waste and pointless treatment.

Kenneth Clarke's reforms in the early 1990s moved in that direction. His was a flanking movement. Knowing full well that ripping up the catechism of the NHS, which featured 'free at the point of delivery' as the first commandment, was a bridge too far, Ken's strategy was stealthy, placing GPs in charge of budgets on behalf of patients instead. The results of even this limited reform were remarkable: prescription budgets of pioneering practices were cut by 25 per cent; where control extended to emergency admissions, cost reductions of up to 40 per cent were achieved; and new facilities, developed from the savings in response to the patient's desire to have simple procedures performed closer to home and on demand, blossomed.

Third party payments also encourage unnecessarily high healthcare costs. The first problem is overuse and inappropriate use of medical services by patients. From GP surgeries stacked with victims of the common cold for which over the counter remedies are easily available, through ambulance services abused by callers as an alternative taxi service, to the politically correct and cruel maintenance of life of the obviously dying in intensive care units, the spectrum of NHS health care provision is straddled by examples of expensive misuse.

'Excessive' has a well-defined meaning in economics as applied to healthcare – when the marginal value of resources used in treatment is greater than the marginal value derived by the patient from treatment. Used in a purely medical context 'excessive' means treatment which in the opinion of a third party provider, usually distant from the patient – perhaps a health authority, a private insurer, or in a national context the National Institute for Clinical Excellence, (NICE), now guarding the gate of entry to NHS reimbursement, rationing expensive new treatments and drugs – is unneeded. The current debate over 'excessive' use of cesarean sections illustrates the point well. But value in the eye of a remote and bureaucratic third party with sights fixed firmly on national budgets may not be value in the eyes of the patient.

In other areas of life we happily get on with deciding what we need on our own, or, when expert help is needed, turn to specialists who buy services on our behalf. An airline ticket may be bought on the web, but for a tour up the Amazon a travel agent will be consulted. The guardians of the NHS flame respond by claiming health is a singular exception. It is a *de haut en bas* argument, implying that people who are perfectly capable of organising every other aspect of their complex lives, housing, nutrition, bringing up families, working as tradesmen, professionals, Health Secretaries, whatever, draw a blank when it comes to healthcare.

Having lost that argument the guardians turn to another myth, that we need an NHS to provide healthcare equally across the population. Never mind that in 50 years of the NHS that has never been achieved, the suggestion is that with a bit more effort the creaking, centralised system will deliver. If it could not deliver equality in the straightforward 1950's it certainly will not in the increasingly complex world that is twenty-first century healthcare.

Would handing patients the purse strings make a difference?

What is the point of focussing purchasing power on the patient? As Jonathan Reggler notes elsewhere in this book, in the 1980s the Rand Corporation in the US carried out the most extensive research ever conducted into third party payment mechanisms for healthcare. It observed how different forms of co-payment for medical services affected the behaviour of 2,500 families for a period of 3–5 years. They were divided into groups ranging from Group A, whose medical expenses were totally reimbursed by a third party insurer, to Group D, who paid 95 per cent of costs. The difference in healthcare usage across the groups was dramatic. Group A used 53 per cent percent more hospital services (measured in cash) than Group D and 63 per cent more usage of visits to doctors, consumption of drugs and the like. The point at which behaviour changed markedly was when co-payments for services exceeded 50 per cent of the cost.

Should we be surprised that an analysis of the health outcomes of these groups showed not a whit of variation between those who had splurged other people's money and those who had spent, on average, 58 per cent less of their own? It proved that big spending does not necessarily equate with better health outcomes.

Cut waste

One fortuitous impact of shifting the responsibility for funding to consumers would be on wasteful spending. A self-imposed control on expensive technical, medical and therapeutic interventions whose value is often illusory would secure savings. Today the NHS is a patsy for every shiny piece of kit, wonder drug or screening process that can rally a pressure group to its cause on the *Today* programme. Breast screening is a popular feminist cause, carried out at huge public expense, but with dubious benefits. No critic dares say so.

The media plays shamelessly on the susceptibility of families with children who need pioneering, unproven surgery unavailable on the NHS, but deliverable in Houston, Texas. The battle is now a familiar set piece: create scandal that the NHS can't deliver; tearful family bemoans 'lack of resources'; government of the day condemned as uncaring; media organises whip round; sends unfortunate child to Houston; then, usually silence as the answer to that awkward question, 'did it work?' is more often than not, in the negative.

Don't despair – two solutions

Ending the system of third party payments in the UK by giving patients responsibility for healthcare spending could be achieved in either of two ways. This essay points the direction and is not intended to offer a turnkey solution.

The superficially more acceptable, but on analysis less desirable, proposition is a system of co-payments, as used in the

Rand Corporation trial and practised in other healthcare systems, notably the French. The drawback is that reimbursement for the less well off would require a wasteful paper chase.

To reach the level of effectiveness determined by Rand would also require patients to find significant funds from their own budgets before treatment, accompanied by adverse headlines when patients could not find the cash. Suggestions that nominal charges for GP visits – £5 – would have an impact on demand or the shape of the service offered patients are simply ridiculous. Token gestures will not work.

A more radical approach is needed to give patients sufficient economic clout to promote change. Patients could be 'endowed' at birth with their own healthcare fund, from which they would draw as needs arose. The incentive to use the fund wisely would rest on the principle that on reaching benchmarks defined by age, say 20, 40, 60 and 80, any under-drawn surplus could be returned to the patient directly. Cash would be the most powerful incentive, but if that were too crude for polite public taste, a pension top up would be a possible alternative.

Is it not impossible to define the size of the fund? In spite of all the trials and tribulations of the NHS and its seemingly unpluggable demand for more cash, the DoH has a sound actuarial grip on the average healthcare needs of UK citizens in cash terms, over their lifetimes. Mr or Mrs UK consumes the bulk of healthcare spending during the first six and the last three years of life. For the rest of an average lifetime the spending graph is flat, except for the small minority affected by traumatic injury or the onset of chronic disease. The fund would be reassessed to reflect the impact of inflation on, say, a five yearly basis.

What if the fund runs out? It is not beyond the wit of healthcare policy makers to define areas of high cost care, which would not impact upon the fund. Emergency trauma and chronic illness are the two obvious examples.

How would the patient use the fund? Initially, spending would be through a GP of the patient's choice, a logical extension of the fund-holding principle that delivered such rapid innovation in care provision and improvements in patient service during the 1990s. Over time, perhaps speciality hospitals would offer quality care for elective procedures, like heart surgery, where outcomes are largely determined by a high volume of throughput. A patient could make the choice between hospitals and surgeons who would have to attract business on price and quality rather than relying on local gossip and bed-side manner, and perhaps pay more to be treated more quickly. Hospitals which failed to deliver services patients wanted would lose funds and be forced to change, or close. That was what the internal market of Kenneth Clarke's reforms was beginning to achieve before its teeth were drawn by Labour.

Perhaps patients would choose not to deplete the fund at all for certain treatments. Instead of a £50 visit to the GP, a trip to the chemist for a £5 over the counter remedy might be a more sensible option.

Investment in new high cost technology and pharmaceuticals would not be driven by pressure groups or industry self interest but by questions rarely heard in the NHS today, 'How will the patient value this and will I receive a return on my investment?'

Preventive and, perhaps, novel therapies

In 1948 it was fondly thought that the NHS would make people more healthy. Instead, all it has done is treat the sick. Preventive healthcare has always been the Cinderella of the service because there was nothing in it for patients. Moralistic lectures to Glaswegians about the cardiac risk incurred by wolfing deep-fried, batter-encrusted, Mars Bars have always fallen on deaf ears. Year after year of gloomy anti-smoking ads have resulted in the highest levels of female teenage smoking ever. Increased risk is admitted, but rarely personalised. Saving cash by maintaining good health is a sharper, more easily understood proposition. Why not allow repayments from the fund for those who meet a number of 'good health' indicators, as insurance companies offer discounted policies for non-smokers today?

There is an arrogant assumption among many medical practitioners that their branch of medicine should enjoy monopoly access to public funds. There is erosion at the margins as primary care begins to allocate small chunks of budget to alternative care, especially as outcomes data emerges from studies of homeopathic remedies that puts some products on a par with conventional pharmaceutical products for effectiveness. Often alternative remedies are less toxic than conventional equivalents, a point that may weigh heavily with an informed patient. The bulk of budgets are held by the medical establishment, which pooh-pooh's any attack on its citadel by 'outsiders,' so locating the power of the budget at a different level would be a catalyst for change.

Will it ever happen?

The public is in the mood for a debate about a radical change in healthcare funding, even if the government and the Conservative opposition, whose only policy on health seems to be to say 'me too' as fast as possible to higher spending, is not.

The mission of Mr Derek Wanless, to look with a radical eye at the NHS so long as he doesn't even speculate on how it is funded, is 'Mission Impossible'. What is even more absurd is the politicians' eagerness – and this a cross-party *folie* – to keep holding a hot potato that has scorched the hands of every Health Secretary and Minister who has gingerly held it since 1948.

There are many areas of life where the state needs to step in to supply a national need. Healthcare is no longer one of them. The state has a proper role as guarantor of standards and watchful guardian of patients' rights of access. As the budget holder and provider of care it is now out of its depth in an area where a lumbering centralised bureaucracy is unable to respond to rapid changes in clinical practice, the introduction of potentially cost effective technology and therapies and limitless patient demand. Forget pious bleating about policy documents on 'patients' rights', give them the greatest right of all, control of the cash that funds the healthcare they need.

Healthcare in the UK: where do we go from here?

Ruth Lea

Introduction

The current state of the NHS should concern us all – including the business community. An efficient healthcare system is as much a part of the country's infrastructure (as well as being a mark of a civilised society) for a thriving business sector as is the transport system and education. It seems so obvious and yet, to my knowledge, business organisations have been remarkably reticent on health matters.

Sickness is, of course, a major cost for business and, if an employee goes long term sick, this can be very disruptive, especially for small businesses. Businesses have to keep jobs open for sick people – unless they feel the situation is so unsustainable that they dismiss the person on grounds of lack of capability (and then risk charges of unfair dismissal). In addition, delayed and cancelled appointments add to business's burdens as well as being very unpleasant for the employee in question. Moreover, corporate health insurance is not so much a perk these days, as a necessary part of the remuneration package for some employees. Business may well ask why they pay their taxes and then have to provide health insurance for employees.

It was with these (and other more personal) thoughts in mind that I originally wrote my report *Healthcare in the UK: the need for reform.*[1] It was, on my part, a modest attempt to stimulate a debate on the nature of the NHS and the need for, non-ideological, reform. Moreover, it didn't claim to be able to 'solve' the NHS's problems overnight. With the current difficulties of the NHS apparently mounting by the week, the need for reform grows ever more necessary. But, at least, the debate is now moving ahead. When I wrote my original paper, the reaction was deafening in its silence. Now every one seems to be jumping on the NHS reform bandwagon. But better late than never.

UK healthcare: the problem of 'triple nationalisation'

The fundamental problem is that healthcare in the UK suffers from a 'triple nationalisation' and, therefore, very little competition and, hence, responsiveness to the patient in the system. Moreover, no number of DoH consultations will solve the endemic managerial and cultural problems in the NHS – the last of our late 1940s nationalised industries, a lumbering leviathan, and a highly politicised one at that.

By 'triple nationalisation' we mean:

- *There is a public sector 'quasi-monopoly' of funding.* There is currently a need for more funding – a need that will continue as patient expectations continue to rise and treatments become ever more sophisticated. The 'funding gap' between the UK and the main continental European countries is particularly pronounced in the private rather than the public sector and ways need to be found to incentivise private sector contributions. We recommend a 'passport' scheme which is a type of economic voucher scheme;

- *A public sector 'quasi-monopoly' of decision making about resource allocation*, with the consequence that resources are frequently allocated for 'political' (and 'politically correct') reasons rather than for economic (subsuming health) reasons. Those conditions that are glamorous (appealing to doctors) and have vocal interest groups (for example, AIDS and women's cancers) tend to receive more funding than unglamorous conditions (the elderly and the mentally ill). The politicisation of resource allocation must stop;
- *A public sector 'quasi-monopoly' of healthcare provision and a lack of competition in the healthcare sector*. The absence of competition serves patients poorly; there are few incentives for producers to respond to patient preferences (despite the exhortations in the NHS Plan[2]). We believe that there is a good case for building up the private sector to increase competition (and indeed the public sector's use of private sector facilities) and drive up public sector standards. But, in addition to this, we would convert current public sector provision (which is virtually unmanageable and far too politicised) into private, independent and non-profit making 'mutuals' or alternative not-for-profit models.

I now will consider these three main themes in turn.

Healthcare funding: introduction

There is no doubt that there are now large spending increases in the pipeline for the NHS. Spending was £35bn in 1997/98 and the last Comprehensive Spending Review[3] (CSR) – which covered 2001/02 to 2003/04 and was released in July 2000 – planned nearly £50bn spending for the current financial year (2001/02)[4] and further increases were pencilled in for the subsequent two financial years. Moreover, it is clear that additional spending increases will be announced in forthcoming months, to be paid for, according to the Prime Minister, by higher taxes. (this essay was written in February 2002, before the April Budget and the Summer 2002 CSR, which will cover 2003/04–2005/06, and so the author does not know exactly what these figures will turn out to be.) The Prime Minister's game plan, in particular, seems to be to meet the EU average, though this is fraught with difficulties, not least because it is a moving target.

But even with these increases, whatever they turn out to be, healthcare in the UK will probably still look under-funded by international standards. It is difficult to obtain exactly comparable data but we spend around 7 per cent of GDP (about 6 per cent public sector, 1 per cent private sector) on health compared with 8½ per cent in the Netherlands, 9½ per cent in France, over 10 per cent in Germany and nearly 13 per cent in the US. In particular, our level of private spending is especially low by international standards.

Even though some analysts claim that our outcomes in terms of life expectancy are comparable to other countries and, therefore, the spending gap 'doesn't matter', there is undoubted evidence of a significant 'effectiveness gap' in the treatment of serious diseases including cancer, coronary heart disease (CHD) and stroke between the UK and most other developed countries. Moreover, there is increasing dissatisfaction with, for example, the NHS's waiting times, cleanliness standards, care of the elderly and dealing with chronic non-life threatening problems. Few people are as unquestioningly supportive of the NHS as they were twenty years ago – not least because deference is fading and expectations are rising. Indeed, though there is still sympathy and support for healthcare professionals, there is widespread dissatisfaction with the NHS.

Funding levels *do* need to be reconsidered (and, of course, the supply side needs to be reformed – see below). But even if we just aspired to reaching around 8½ to 9 per cent of GDP on healthcare, we would be looking for considerable extra funding. More specifically, we would be looking for an extra £15–£20bn (some 6–8p on the basic rate of income tax).

We do not believe that putting taxes up by this amount is politically feasible – even though we are being softened up by the Prime Minister to pay more tax. It is so clear that demand will continue to outstrip publicly funded supply – especially as the population is ageing, treatments are getting more expensive, increasingly non-deferential 'consumerist' patients become more demanding and, according to latest reports, our 'couch potato society' will produce more sick people. The situation is grave now. We fear that it will get worse. There is, therefore, a need to consider incentivising more private sector funding and, though I would not regard this as quite so urgent a matter as trying to reform the provision side, at some point, I suggest, it will have to be tackled.

Funding: the 'NHS passport'

There are several approaches to significantly increasing funding. Briefly they are:

- Extra **income taxes** (whether hypothecated or not). As we've already suggested, we do not believe this is politically feasible in the long-term;
- A **social insurance scheme** as in many continental countries. We see three major problems. Firstly, it would be a step change for the UK and, therefore, could be difficult to introduce; secondly, much of the cost burden could fall on employers and, thirdly, such schemes don't necessarily respond well to individual 'wants';
- Significantly extending **PMI**. But we accept the well-rehearsed problems with PMI (cherry picking, adverse selection, complex contracts with extensive exclusions etc) and feel that, whilst it undoubtedly has its place, it isn't much of a runner for major extra funding;
- **Increased charges**. But there would need to be extensive exemptions and, therefore, would be unlikely to raise much revenue. Not the way forward.

To solve these problems our preferred approach is the **'NHS Passport' scheme** (an economic voucher scheme).

In this scheme:

- Each person would have an 'NHS Passport' which would entitle him/her to 'core services' that are **free at the point of access** and would be funded by the taxpayer as at present. There would be no limitations on the person's access to core services. Use would be determined by clinical need;

- The core services would be strictly defined (with the types of treatment available also strictly defined) and concentrate on serious and long-term illness and packages of care for certain groups including babies, children, pregnant women and the elderly;
- If the patient wished to use NHS facilities for core services, their treatment would be free;
- If the patient wished to use other, private sector, facilities for core services they would be given a 'credit note' (a voucher) to the value (necessarily conservatively estimated) of their NHS funded treatment and pay the marginal cost or 'top up' charge. We feel this would enable people to use private sector treatment more easily ('why should they pay twice through their taxes to the NHS and directly to the private sector?') and stimulate competition. In addition, if they wished to use NHS provision but wanted an expensive drug not yet approved for NHS 'core treatment' they would pay the marginal cost, not the total cost;
- If the patient wished to have treatment for non-core services, they would pay the whole cost. The NHS would, *de facto*, be drawing back from the notion that it can be or indeed should be 'free and comprehensive' (though, in reality, it is not totally free at the point of use now, nor is it fully comprehensive). People may baulk at this – but, if a tax-payer funded NHS is to be feasible in the medium-term some very hard choices will have to be taken. And the passport system, which after all refunds some money to the patient if he/she goes private, would simply not be financially viable.

NHS: resource allocation

The second of our 'triple nationalisations' concerns resource allocation.

NHS resources are currently frequently allocated for 'political' reasons, with an unacceptable lack of transparency, rather than for economic (subsuming clinical) reasons. 'Glamorous' conditions, which appeal to doctors and researchers and/or have vocal interest groups (e.g. AIDS and women's cancers), tend to receive relatively more funding than 'unglamorous' conditions (e.g. the elderly and the mentally ill). The politicisation of resource allocation should stop. Of course, AIDS and women's cancers should be treated – but so should the elderly and the mentally ill.

We feel that there should be a public debate concerning what should be included in the core services – the National Institute for Clinical Excellence (NICE) is well suited to lead such a debate. We have noticed a marked reluctance by many people to grasp this nettle. But we believe it is a nettle that has to be grasped. The alternative is the current system of rationing by delay (waiting lists), denial (no treatment at all) or dilution (second best treatment)[5]. Rationing is, to use the vernacular, 'big' in the NHS. As part of the debate, the notion of maximising economic 'health gain' (subject to the very necessary condition of respecting the autonomy of the individual) should be central. Any treatments that are unsatisfactory in economic terms (which subsumes clinical effectiveness) should be ruled out. We would concentrate resources on serious and long-term illness and packages of care for certain groups (babies, children, pregnant women and the elderly). IVF and confessional counselling, for example, would not be in core services.

Moreover, much of the **health promotion advice**, as propagated in the Public Health White Papers *Health of the Nation* (1992) and *Saving Lives: Our Healthier Nation* (1999), would fail to make the grade. Our analysis showed that much of it was not based on sound science (the standard advice on alcohol consumption, for example, is ludicrous: if it were really true I and most of my friends would be dead). It should be quietly dropped and replaced by common sense from the doctor!

Turning to **screening**, the current programmes for women (breast cancer and cervical cytology) are both remarkably ineffective and very dishonest[5] – especially cervical screening. They are both expensive (especially cervical screening as GPs are financially incentivised to meet targets), they both throw up a large number of false 'positives' and both 'save' remarkably few lives. Breast screening may save one life in every 3,000 mammograms, according to the latest data, but it throws up a 5 per cent chance of a 'positive' result, of which over 90 per cent are 'false'. Cervical screening may save one life in every 5,000 smear tests (falling to, say, one in 50,000 for low risk groups), but it throws up a 6 per cent chance of a 'positive' result, of which 98–99 per cent are 'false'.[6] And then there are 'false negatives' which can delay correct diagnosis and treatment. These screening programmes would not be in core services. The resources currently dedicated to these programmes would be far better allocated to treatment, including cancer treatment where there is a shortage of funds. To misallocate resources in healthcare, as happens with women's cancer screening, is irresponsible. You lose lives in the system.

NHS: provision

The third 'triple nationalisation' concerns the provision or supply side. Change here is, we suggest, the top priority. Without reform in delivery we can have little chance of any significant improvements in the NHS.

Our NHS 'passport' entitles people to free core services. But who is to provide the services? Well, it most certainly doesn't need to be the NHS in its current form with its patient-insensitive, near-monopoly of healthcare provision and its consequent lack of competition. (The lack of competition, incidentally, disadvantages doctors and other healthcare professionals as well as patients because a proper market cannot function for their skills.) It is vital that a more competitive market is developed for healthcare. Moreover, the NHS, with its million employees and huge budgets, is an unmanageable leviathan. The NHS is the last of the monopolistic nationalisations and, very obviously, a political football.

Competitive pressures are by far the best way of making a system sensitive and responsive to patients' preferences. The current approach of bombarding NHS staff with a stream of politicised 'management' initiatives (most of which probably wouldn't see the light of day in the private sector) is very much a second best strategy. Moreover, the politically driven 'permanent revolution' of organisational changes saps energy and enthusiasm and results in corrosive cynicism. Provision must be taken out of the political domain. And how to stimulate competition? Well, our NHS passport scheme with its concept of the 'credit note' would undoubtedly help. But we do feel that more is needed.

In my original paper, I constructed a model for healthcare delivery, a 'managed competition' system, along the following lines:

- The NHS would cease being a major provider of care. **The NHS would be redefined as the funder of core services free at the point of access (funded by the taxpayer and accountable to Parliament), which would be decided apolitically, and be the regulator;**
- NHS Trusts for both acute care and community/primary care would become independent non-profit making mutuals. They would not be state owned, they would manage their business affairs independently and be depoliticised;
- These NHS Trusts would comprise the NHS's 'approved' list of providers of core services ('NHS approved Trusts') and be obliged to provide the core services without charge;
- The GPs (now structured within Primary Care Trusts) would remain as gatekeepers to the taxpayer funded core services and fairly strict ones at that;
- The NHS (and its regional offices) would be the conduit for taxpayers' funds for core services;

- The NHS would be the regulator, ensuring that standards were maintained throughout the whole of the healthcare sector (including all the current private and/or voluntary hospitals and clinics), with the Health Authorities and/or the Commission for Health Improvement (CHI or CHIMP) probably taking the lead;
- **And, most importantly of all, provision, along with resource allocation, would be depoliticised.**

Since I wrote my original paper, and at risk of sounding complacent, I haven't felt any need fundamentally to change our broad approach. If anything, I have become more convinced that it is a sensible and positive route to explore and we have, accordingly, developed our ideas, especially on mutuals, further.[7] Mutualising the Trusts could, we suggest, be a strong stimulus to improving top-down management of doctors and other staff within hospitals (some are simply not managed at present) – blessedly free from political interference and the latest 'initiative' from the DoH.

In addition, the general debate on provision has developed quite beyond my wildest expectations.[8] One interesting development is that of Public Interest Companies (PICs)[9] as a possible delivery vehicle for public services including healthcare.

Conclusion

The UK has fallen behind the standards of provision in other developed countries, and it shows. So where do we go from here? Well, I see no alternative to radical reform, which involves over the next decade:

- **Healthcare funding:** people must be incentivised to contribute more to their own healthcare. The idea that the taxpayer should pick up most of the bill for healthcare in all its many forms, though seemingly supported by the current Government, is not, I suggest, viable in the longer term. We do, however, strongly believe that carefully defined 'core services' should be funded by the taxpayer and be delivered free at the point of access. An NHS 'passport' should be available to all – for both taxpayer funded care and private sector care;
- **NHS: resource allocation**: 'core services' should be carefully defined and resources must be allocated on sound economic/clinical principles and not for political (and 'politically correct') reasons. The current system is riddled with rationing – it's time to rationalise the system so people know what they can realistically expect to be funded by the NHS;
- **NHS: provision**: the provision of healthcare services must be taken out of the politicised vice grip of the state. And the NHS, a lumbering leviathan of one million employees, should be broken into more manageable units. Consideration should be given to converting the NHS Trusts into mutuals, which should stimulate top-down management of doctors and other staff free of political interference. The reform of provision is top priority.

---

1 Lea, Ruth: *Healthcare in the UK: the need for reform* (IoD February 2000, revised June 2000). A short 4 page introduction to the full paper is available – also entitled *Healthcare in the UK: the need for reform* (IoD October 2000). See also Lea, Ruth: 'Healthcare in the UK: the need for reform' (*The Business Economist*, Volume 32/1, 2001).

2 NHS: *The NHS Plan: a plan for investment, a plan for reform* (TSO, 2000).

3 HM Treasury: *Spending Review 2000: new public spending plans 2001–2004. Prudent for a purpose: building opportunity and security for all* (TSO, 2000, Cm 4807).

4 See *Daily Telegraph* leader: 'Sick logic' (*Daily Telegraph*, 22 February 2002) which said that spending increases were not resulting in equivalent performance improvements. One reason probably reflects the rapid fluctuations in funding. The NHS was starved of funds in the first 2 years (following the Tories' 'plans', which the Tories would not have stuck to) and switching on the tap after such starvation is fraught with difficulties. NHS provision is still being restricted by serious supply constraints in both medical personnel and physical facilities and a combination of rapidly increasing budgets with supply constraints is a recipe for waste.

5 Green, David, and Casper, Laura: *Delay, Denial and Dilution* (IEA, January 2000).

6 Lea, Ruth: 'Women's cancer screening: time for some honesty' (*British Journal of Health Care*, August 2001).

7 Day, Geraint: *Management, mutuality and risk: better ways to run the National Health Service* (IoD, 2000). *And* Day, Geraint: *Healthcare Provision Policy Study Group: Report of a survey of views on healthcare provision* (IoD, 2001).

8 See, for example Alan Millburn's speech to the New Health Network (15 January 2002), which discussed the possibility of exploring mutualisation or PICs for delivering healthcare. A very important speech.

9 Public Management Foundation (PMF): 'The case for the Public Interest Company: a new form of enterprise for public service delivery' (PMF, June 2001).

Safe in *whose* hands?

Effective consumer power in health care.

Professor John Spiers

In 1948 the NHS abolished the individual customer. Its endemic and intractable problems were thus set in place with its foundation stones. I will argue here that only individual empowerment and control over a personal health care fund will provide the direct incentives to resolve the systemic snags of the NHS.

Consumer empowerment can uniquely broaden the funding base, enhance access, and improve outcomes. It can help us attain an equitable, accessible, reliable and affordable system of care and a different way of seeing ourselves. Consumer choice, also, concerns a broader accountability than that of professionals and providers. It concerns the accountability of consumers themselves to make cost-conscious, cost-effective choices, balancing risk and benefit.

It is a choice between paternalism and preference. As Colin Thubron has said, 'A traveller needs to believe in the significance of where he is, and therefore in his own meaning.'[1] But NHS service-users have had little or no influence on what happens to them in healthcare. This is the case despite the fact that they have seen their individual power over their lives grow in almost every other area of existence. Money talks, and preference walks. We have relied on markets in every area save for some which matter most: health and education. The system is constructed, instead, so that 'experts' can know and provide for our 'needs'.

The NHS has substituted collectiv*ism* for collective (voluntary) action. In the bureaucratised state monopoly system individuals have had no individual economic power by which to signal their wishes, wants, and preferences. Instead, various 'expert agents' – Ministers of the Crown, Civil Servants, GPs, Health Authorities, Primary Care Trusts, and 'representative' bodies – have decided on their 'needs' on their behalf. They have assumed it is possible to second-guess the wishes of others. If this approach was applied to our food or our shelter we would be outraged. Yet these are more fundamental even than our health. In post-war Britain much credit is due to the tides of progress in liberal capitalist society. These have improved living standards, diet, housing, leisure, travel, and the quality of life. The poor and the disadvantaged have been aided and able to function in markets, to their own and the general advantage. Yet in healthcare the poor have done least well, with no bargaining power. transferring signals about preferences and willingness to pay. But in the NHS these key externals have been suppressed.

Since self-responsible choice and competition were constrained the NHS was wholly politicised from day one. Voting and 'consultation' has proved no substitute for choice and competition. Indeed, the key point at the heart of this debate is that the option of being enabled to *discipline* a system by an occasional vote or a sporadic consultation, is not the same as an individual being able to *command* a personal service when, where, and from whom they want it. And this is a fundamental deficit, for, of all aspects of our humanity, our health care is intimate, personal, specific, differentiated, and reliant on timely and appropriate services.

We need to understand, however, that politicians are as much prisoners of the existing structure as are ordinary service-users. Max Weber said that man is an animal suspended in webs of significance he himself has spun. The iconic status of the NHS makes prisoners of us all, ministers included. Perhaps the most important constraint on reality, present, and future is this 'prison of awe'. However, we are at last seeing wider discussion of the idea that the NHS is not the *only* possibility, and that alternatives in place elsewhere actually deliver proven better care. Mr Alan Milburn, Secretary of State for Health, has changed many things. He has shown courage in facing issues previously ignored, such as the individual performance records of doctors.[2] But the changes he is sponsoring themselves reveal the logical contradictions which will not permit financially-empowered consumer choice within a state monopoly system.

I suggest that the only credible resolution of these apparently intractable difficulties lies in effective and financially-empowered individual choice and self-responsibility. Empowerment brings ourselves, our actions, our responsibilities, our expectations sharply into the light. It also focuses us, too, on what the NHS has achieved, where it has fallen short, and why. And, the

Political academic Jeremy Shearmur has reminded us of the importance of correcting our theories 'rather than suffering the consequences of action on the basis of false theories: of allowing our theories to die in our stead.'[3]

In the contrast between voting and the voucher, or between consultation and command, we see the fundamental distinction between 'needs' and 'wants'. As Shirley Robin Letwin wrote:

> The NHS was designed to satisfy 'needs' rather than 'wants'. 'Needs' are given by nature, and only experts, doctors and social scientists can know how to satisfy them. Therefore, the patient is to be seen not as a consumer, deciding what he wants, but as a passive recipient of whatever the all-knowing powers on high decide that he ought to have. Therefore consumer sovereignty would defeat the purpose of a national health service . . . [the organisation] aimed to treat passive bundles of 'needs' rather than independent consumers with a will to choose what they wanted and a right to complain about how their wants were being satisfied.'[4]

The concept of 'needs' contradicts the self-responsibility implied by the word 'wants'. Its partners in this burglary of the patients' rights are both ageism and a gender-biased service.[5] Its frame of mind is refluxed in the advocacy of the virtues of allocative rationing by many academics and administrators opposed to individual empowerment and committed to health care for 'populations'. This, too, despite the evidence to the contrary from almost all OECD members and from an important recent study of Kaiser Permanente in America.[6]

Thus, empowerment is not a marginal add-on, which will somehow 'sensitise' monopoly providers and somehow re-balance the picture without changing the frame. It is not another way of 'representing' consumers as one 'interest' among many. I suggest it is *the* key, *the* unique, *the* irresistible lever to help break up the triple-nationalisation and quasi-monopolies of funding, purchasing/rationed allocation, and provision. There is a vital point here, too, about the nature of modern care and the necessity of empowerment. Without patient empowerment, confident self-knowledge, more self-care and personal responsibility, the advantageous shift from institutional to domiciliary settings cannot be achieved. We need to endorse the principles of empowerment, whichever financially-empowering device is chosen to effect these changes.[7]

There is a real sense, however, in which people have voted themselves poor healthcare, by clinging to the idea that this can somehow be 'free'. And that it is best provided (overseas evidence to the contrary) by a state monopoly based on limited tax revenues, with quasi-monopoly purchasing and provision. Meanwhile, the state disables what markets uniquely enable: price-conscious choice in a competitive market, the personal ability to increase spending in response to preferences, the evolution of more (and more responsive) provision, notably from private sources. This burdens many with unnecessary suffering. In terms of outcomes – by comparison with the many of the 29 OECD partner countries – our record concerning patient survival from serious disease, poorer life quality (especially among elderly sufferers from chronic conditions) and longevity has been weaker than it might have been in a system of voluntary exchange. We are continuing to fall behind the quality and access to services *routinely* expected in other advanced countries.[8] What may have seemed to be freedom from payment has, indeed, produced a general condemnation to services below the minimum acceptable in other advanced countries. The NHS remains outside the modern incentive-based service economy.

The assumptions the NHS embodies.

The pivotal question is who decides who decides? Here Sir Isaiah Berlin, in *Four Essays on Liberty*, maps the territory. He shows us what kind of approach to liberty the NHS represents, and what we should instead seek. Berlin says:

> There are two separate questions. One is 'How many doors are open to me?'; the other is: 'Who is in control?' These questions are interwoven, but they are not the same, and they require different answers. How many doors are open to me? The question about the extent of negative liberty is to do with what obstacles lie before me. What am I prevented from doing by other people – deliberately or indirectly, unintentionally or institutionally? The other question is 'Who governs me? Do others govern me or do I govern myself? If others, by what right, what authority? If I have a right to self-rule, autonomy, can I lose this right? Can I give it away? Waive it? Recover it? In what way? Who makes the laws? Or implements them? Am I consulted? Does the majority govern? Why? Does God? The priests? The Party? The pressure of public opinion? Or tradition? By what authority?

> Both questions, and their sub-questions, are central and legitimate. Both have to be answered.... Both are genuine questions. Both are inescapable. And the answers to them determine the nature of a given society.'[9]

We can see that we must privilege and protect 'negative liberty', or the freedom to be ourselves. The individual must be trusted to make decisions we might not make for ourselves.

Meanwhile, the assumptions represented by the NHS show us several denials at once.

First, by substituting 'expert' guidance for individual choice the NHS represents *a fundamental misunderstanding about the nature of knowledge*, and of what we can know of another. Even, of what we can know, in advance, about our own selves, prior to actually having to make a difficult decision when faced, for example, with serious illness.

The model does not recognise the severe limits to the possibility of knowledge about the preferences of others – let alone limits on how this often tacit (and socially divided) knowledge can be centralised. It relies on the idea that an expert can know someone else's good, or 'needs' better than they can for themselves. This denial of choice is based on the idea that there are knowable 'needs' and specific outcomes which politicians and 'experts' can and should know, and which can somehow be captured in 'policy'. That experts can decide on what should be acceptable quality for many diverse individuals, how high quality can and should be, and on the priority listing of who should be treated first, and who last or not at all.[10] This belief assumes that human values and preferences can be derived from some understandings about human nature, and what all want. Indeed, that all want the same things, and that these are not in conflict. Berlin has shown us that this is not the case, in his discussion of 'incommensurables'. Karl Popper (and after him, Robert Nozick) also concluded that liberty and material equality were incompatible. The increasing diversity of our society underlines the point.[11]

Second, the denial of choice is based on the idea that *government should decide what it is appropriate for the individual to spend* on health care, where and how money should be 'allocated' or 'targeted', usually in the interests of a political objective such as 'equality'.

Third, the state monopoly *encourages misunderstandings about the character of much healthcare*. In fact, healthcare is a commodity concerning life-style choices more often than it is a crisis buy concerning life or death decisions. And even when the individual faces serious disease, personal preferences about the outcomes an individual can live with are fundamental. Indeed, where the choice is how to live with a disease which the individual can survive for 5, 10, or more years, these life-style choices are paramount. Yet a consumer good has been confused with welfare. Personal choice is, in fact, crucial in self-management to benefit from treatments.

Disempowerment of the poor is not, either, the result of markets. It is instead significantly (but not wholly) due to the suppression of market signals and the lack of income provided to them from tax-transfers to enable them to secure better access to quality health care. Health economist Robert Evans has shown, too, that much disease is an *expression* of other non-medical factors. Self-esteem is a vital factor in good health, in feeling in control of one's own life, of being an effective actor in choices. Empowerment can renovate self-esteem, by fortifying demand with tax-money in individual hands so that consumers predominate over providers, and with incentives to pursue personal goals by leading any increase in private spending on health care. Meanwhile, the poor die earlier, and from otherwise treatable disease. They experience a disproportionate share of disease and suffering and pain. Since good health is recognised as one of the rewards of economic and social power, of education and understanding, we must make efforts to empower the poor with tax-transfers so that they can function effectively in competitive markets.[12]

Can the NHS empower the service-user?

There is now much fashionable talk of making [*sic*] the NHS consumer-friendly. Of increasing the 'involvement' and 'consultation' of patients, on 'priority setting' and other issues bureaucracies select. However, these initiatives tellingly demonstrate the limits of possible reform within the politicised and bureaucratised system.

There are three approaches to empowering the individual. First, that of centralism, where government supports professionals to make decisions: 'positive liberty', or empowerment of others but for our own good. This approach – aside from its moral and ethical defects – has given very poor results in terms of avoidable disease, outcomes and longevity. It gives no ultimate sanctions to the individual, even if good practitioners do much to help individuals make informed choices. The second approach is that of seeking to 'sensitise' services to users' views with a multiplicity of mechanisms for 'listening' to local people, together with devolution to local institutions. But this programme offers no specific accountability to the individual, and no individual leverage. It merely shifts power into local versions of central control. The third approach is consumerist. It financially empowers the individual by re-distributing power itself.

These approaches represent incompatible alternatives by which consumers can try to express preferences. Let us look at centralist ideas for empowerment.

First, look at voting. The centralist idea of 'positive liberty' offers accountability by voting. But this is an occasional, often confused and unfocussed way to secure a personal service amongst a bundle of competing issues (Health, Education, Transport, Taxation, Defence, the Euro etc.). The substitution of a political and general choice for individual preference leaves government itself in the irresolvable difficulty of trying to define an 'adequate' service, and the 'right' level of spending. It is impossible to define what healthcare, and in which quantity, the individual should receive.

Trying to command a specific personal service by voting is very different from the daily referendum of empowered personal preference in the market – voting with one's health passport, wallet, voucher, tax-transfer, or secure social insurance right. Only this approach to empowerment can secure self-responsible choices. Here the work of providers is subject to constant check. Meanwhile, one size fits nobody.

Second, look at 'consultation' and 'advocacy' as substitutes for financial empowerment. As consumerism has arisen in society governments have paid obeisance to more consumer control, whilst struggling unavailingly to give back some semblance of power to consumers. The emphasis has been on working with local interests, 'integrating stake-holders' into something called 'the local health economy.' Services have been urged to be more 'responsive', to 'involve consumers', to 'consult' service-users, to have 'more partnership working', to construct 'models of patient-centred care', to 'listen to local voices', and to 'make' the consumer's point of view a priority. Yet it remains a characteristic deficit in Britain that the consumer has no clout.[13]

Instead, we have a profusion of politicised substitutes. This approach has produced a confetti of advisory and executive bodies. A stream of directives, regulatory participation, targets, guidelines, and consultative devices – the panoply and panjandrum of artificial and managed scarcity, centralised allocation, and marginal managerial mellifluousness. These devices must make *some* difference, of course, whether or not they are cost-effective. But when patient push conflicts with political shove, managers are as likely to be sustained in office as to be disciplined by the centre, for political reasons, as we saw in February

2002 when anxiety about Trade Union opposition intruded on the performance management of failing Trusts.[14]

The non-market approach asks for us all to be health activists. Service-users do not exist as players unless they join organised groups, and even then they are merely voices without vouchers. Will Anderson and Steve Gillam have observed that there has been the difficulty 'of enabling a massive state institution, supported by a powerful professional class, to treat its users as consumers, that is, to provide services which are responsive to users needs [sic] and interests.'[15] This implies that only something as powerful as money in the hands of consumers can make the change. And if individuals controlled their own fund, would reform of the NHS take 10 years?

The third substitute for empowerment that is offered is more accountability through local democracy, as advocated by Patrick Jenkin in 1982, and by Simon Jenkins recently.[16] But I think it will be seen that personal choice is not advanced by bringing 'accountability for public spending closer to its consumers through the agencies of local democracy.' Local government may indeed need to be revived, but that is a different political project entirely. We do not want more 'public sector choice', refereed by local 'experts'. This is unlikely to generate individual choice amongst and between public and private providers. If there is to be 'more communal choice' it is essential that this is voluntarily and spontaneously evolved, and that individuals can move their funds if they wish. The entire idea of empowerment by politicised 'consultation' asks more of the service-user than of the provider. It asks the individual to become an activist. Yet few wish to be militant activists, 'helping' to 'decide' the shape of services for the future.

Presently we have no way of assessing how much individuals value health care as a purchase, and of how much additional money they would spend if they could. It is logically incoherent to expect consumer power to emerge within a system of artificial scarcity and central allocation, of a quasi-monopoly of funding, purchasing, and provision. For choice requires extra capacity and the freedom of resources to move to meet expressed preferences. It enjoins the freedom of revenues which prompt new provision. The lack of a significant private provider market restricts the movement of contracts.

Disempowerment of the individual is thus clearly seen as inherent in the existing cultural and political structures and presumptions. These favour the liaison of government, management, and professional interests – Milton Friedman's 'Iron Triangle' – which excludes the service-user.[17] The NHS is, indeed, the classic mirror of the economics of politics studied by James Buchanan, Gordon Tullock, and the 'public choice' economists.[18] It has entrenched centralisation and bureaucracy, because it was built on political assumptions which rejected dynamic user-led evolution. It is these problems which make a patient-focussed service elusive. The patient has no choice, exit, or individual financial clout. There are insufficient revenues to prompt significant new supply. Patient choice without individual, self-responsible financial clout –

and the economic implications of new provision – will remain a chimera.

Is the consumer too ignorant to be empowered?

One argument against individual empowerment has been that consumer ignorance is a fatal bar. But ignorance and the information-assymetry do not arise from the *a priori* character of the irresponsible patient. Ignorance is a *result* of the existing system. There is little or no encouragement to inform oneself, and no leverage if you are informed. The state avoids helping people ask the hard questions, because it allocates from enforced scarcities. However, when consumers have been informed (for example, by the mass media on choices concerning breast cancer treatments) the results have been significant and positive. Consider, too, the following points. First, we do not know what the 'right' choice in any given situation would be. Culture, values, attitudes significantly condition right and wrong choices. So, too, do the uncertainties of medicine itself. Second, education matters, and is essential and constructive. It is specifically prompted by markets, when real choices exist. It was very striking that when Mr Milburn announced that he would publish individual surgeons' heart surgery death rates from April 2004 the British Heart Foundation *immediately* said it would provide counsellors to help patients assess the data.[19] Markets generate information.

Public policy must ensure that consumers are informed, and that they understand the meaning of data and the choices they face. We should notice, too, that no-one ever *really* knows. Medicine is a game of probabilities, and surprises. Much medical care is about judgement, preference, life-style choices, trial and error, and cultural choices. And the impact of medical care itself can be much over-stated.[20]

There are many ghosts which have prevented us facing ourselves. Price, like profit, has been a forbidden word. But it is important to remind ourselves that without price any increase in funding uncovers new unmet demand, which stretches the gap once more. Price is a signal and an incentive or dis-incentive in the unique discovery process of the market. So one key question for any healthcare system is, where do you place price in the system? This is an absolutely fundamental question. At the point of entry into a health plan for the future, by compulsory insurance, or at the point of use? We shall have to face this, for price is the only known effective mechanism for matching demand with supply. And the only known mechanism for setting prices efficiently is a market. This, however, does not mean payment for critical illness interventions at the time of use, though it cannot exclude – save in dream-land – pre-payment, either by taxation or by insurance. We need to grow up, too, with regard to 'profit'. The issue concerning profit from healthcare is not that it must not exist. Even non-profit organisations must recover their costs, pay for their capital, and invest for development. 'Profit' is essential if we are to see investment, and the survival of the best provider. The issue concerning profit is not that we do not want it, but who gets it, and why. In health care it should go to reward good providers, encourage investment, lower costs to consumers, and improve services.

What it would mean for a user-led service to become real rather than rhetorical.

How large is the gap between what we see around us now and what would be necessary for services to be user-led? The tests that rhetoric was converted into reality would include:

1 That users control the agenda, through the cumulative and adaptive power of individual financial decision making. Each consumer would be in charge of a mobile and personal health care fund with which they voluntarily subscribe to a registered insurer and to an approved purchaser which acts on their behalf. Thus, service users (banded together in mutual-aid organisations) would control budgetary allocation and directly influence the ability of providers to secure revenue flows – banded together in mutual-aid organisations. Consumers would have an open choice between competing insurers and providers, and thus between competing doctors, including GPs, and other services, including alternative therapies.

2 That there is price-conscious choice between competing insurers, competing purchasers, and competing providers. Individuals would have the right to review plans at statutory intervals (annually, or every two years) and move if they wish This will ensure consumer bargaining power and the incentive to satisfy wants.

3 That there is meaningful choice, so that consumer can actually access services they wish to have, and incentives to encourage potential providers to come into the market to offer these to willing consumers.

4 That consumers will be free to top-up their individual fund provided through taxation with supplementary insurance, and to negotiate a policy excess which would encourage out-of-pocket payment for small items, and discourage waste. There would be incentives and opportunities to invest above the minimum. And a no-claims bonus could accrue into pension or elderly-care cover. This would be part of the 'guaranteed care package' which government ensures is available to all. Any individual may choose to spend as much more of their own resources on health and social care as they wish. For example, on effective cancer drugs available in continental Europe but denied to patients by the NHS.

5 That users are expected to predominate in decision-making about their own care, with legally-enforceable contracts for services between consumer, insurer, purchaser, and provider.

6 That there are no barriers to information, including performance data on individual practitioners and individual centres of service.

7 That information is made available in such a form and with such promptness that it can become personal knowledge, and is thus available for personal choices and for leverage.

8 That services encourage and equip people (by publishing relevant information) to ask the hard questions, which will make up provider deficits, rather than suppress information which conceals deficits in services.

9 That the narrative experiences of users ('like me') are easily shared between users before they accept treatment – a therapy, a drug, an operation, care from a named individual, in a specific institution. This could include competing High-Street advice centres, some developed from NHS Direct, including support and access to patient groups on the net.

10 That users' own expectations of their roles change, as they assume that it is

reasonable, normal, legitimate, proper to ask for what they want and are ready to pay for, instead of being pre-occupied with guilt.

11 That users themselves decide how much power they are to have, rather than professionals, managers, and politicians deciding how much power to grant them. Here, self-esteem would be strengthened as people feel more in control of their lives, as they are treated as a person and not merely as a 'case'.

12 That people expect to take responsibility for themselves and their families. Thus, choices are rooted in self-jurisdiction, self-responsibility, and a personal assessment of risk, cost-effectiveness, and outcome (responsibly advised by competing advisory services) so that the individual can decide with which situation and outcomes they can live and cope.

13 That surprise, discovery, and learning to choose are welcomed in a framework where government sets the rules but otherwise limits its own role to setting standards, registering medical training, validation and inspection, tax-funding in a diverse funding system, public health initiatives etc.. Government would withdraw to the essential rampart of controlling the framework of rules.

14 That front-line staff have the power to make a difference, and that we realise that money is not the only thing which achieves change. Attitudes, behaviour, communication make a considerable difference to service-users.

15 That as a consequence of these changes creative management, morale, recruitment and retention would improve, as would the rewards for good services. Individual empowerment thus would empower many relationships for constructive change.

For all these things to be real and at the heart of a consumer-led service – indeed, its very axis – we need to see massive cultural shifts in expectations, attitudes, language, and behaviours, by politicians, professionals, and patients too. Indeed, many of these could come about without any extra money, if people changed their attitudes and really got themselves organised. But more money is necessary to prompt new provision, and direct incentives will assure cultural change. When considered from the perspective of such a list, we see, how far we are from individual self-responsibility and from the personalised, consumer-led service which the Secretary of State has set as an objective. Few, if any, believe the modern answers to its difficulties are more politics.

And the answer to the question 'Safe in *whose* hands?' Charles Darwin once said we are 'all netted together'. Social solidarity matters. But we have our own futures in our own hands. As economist Dennis Lees put it, 'The major aim of the liberal is to leave the ethical problem for the individual to wrestle with'[21] If we seek a 'big idea', there is no substitute for an old one.

---

1 Colin Thubron, *In Siberia* (London, Chatto & Windus, 1999).

2 'Milburn unveils his vision for a competitive future', *Health Service Journal*, 25 October 2001; Nicholas Timmins and Rosemary Bennett, 'Private input 'could create new model for hospitals', *Financial Times*, 16 January 2002; Nicholas Timmins, 'Extravagant vision may yield change only at the margins', *Financial Times*, 16 January 2002; Nicholas Timmins, 'A revolution in the NHS', *Financial Times*, 21 January 2002; David Charter and Tom Baldwin, 'NHS consultants to be put under closer scrutiny,' *The Times*, 17 January 2002; Ben Russell, 'Maternity units could be next for the 'league table' treatment, says minister,' *The Independent*, 21 January 2002; Ben Russell, 'Labour plans to overturn principle of free NHS', *The Independent*, 7 February 2002; David Charter and Nigel Hawkes, 'Milburn headhunts entrepreneurs to run failing hospitals', *The Times*, 11 February 2002.

3 Jeremy Shearmur, 'Popper and Classical Liberalism', *Economic Affairs,* Vol.21, No.4, December 2001, pp.37–40.

4 Shirley Robin Letwin, *The Anatomy of Thatcherism* (London, Fontana, 1992), pp.204–5. Examples of this dominant needs-mentality are as common as blackberries. It is regarded as normal, and as invisible as the air we breathe. The language is so pervasive as to be unnoticed, its assumptions so apparently unproblematic as to seem inevitable. But this is not so. See, as an example of assumptions presented as God-given, Jennifer Dixon, 'Transforming the NHS: what chance for the government?', *Economic Affairs,* Vol.21, No.4, December 2001, pp.4–8.

5 David Millward, 'Doctors 'are still writing off patients aged 60 and over'', *Daily Telegraph,* 19 January 2002; Ruth Lea, *Health care in the UK: The Need for Reform* (London, Institute of Directors, 2000).

6 Richard G.A.Feachem, Neelam K.Sekhri, and Karen L.White, 'Getting more for their dollar: a comparison of the NHS with California's Kaiser Permanente', *BMJ,* 2002: 324, pp.135–43; A.C.Enthoven, 'Commentary: Competition made them do it', *BMJ,* 324, 19 January 2002, p.143.

7 The various canvassed devices are comprehensively reviewed by Ruth Lea in *Health care in the UK: The Need for Reform* (London, Institute of Directors, 2000).

8 OECD Electronic Publications, Paris, *OECD Health Data 1998: A Comparative Analysis of 29 Countries*; *OECD Health Data 2001: A Comparative Analysis of 30 Countries* (10th edition). Website: www.oecd.org The OECD is the notary of competing notions about what works best where, the irrefutable corrective of received ideas, partial views, and a priori constructions, despite the difficulties of direct international comparisons. See also Heinz Redwood, *Why Ration Health care? An international study of the United Kingdom, France, Germany and public sector health care in the USA* (London, Civitas, 2000); E.Jabubowski, *Health care Systems in the EU, A Comparative Study. European Parliament Working Paper,* SACO 101/revised. Brussels, European Parliament, 1998; World Health Organisation, *World Health Report 2000* (Geneva, WHO, 2000); R.Freeman, *The Politics of Health in Europe* (Manchester, Manchester University Press, 2000).

9 Isaiah Berlin, *Four Essays On Liberty* (Oxford, Oxford University Press, 1969).

10 Michael Polanyi, in *Personal Knowledge, Towards a Post-Critical Philosophy* (Chicago, University of Chicago Press, 1958), has urged the critical importance of tacit knowledge, which people only articulate within themselves when they face an important decision. And that tacit knowledge is one example of local knowledge, dispersed amongst individuals. It is difficult for planners to gather and interpret this knowledge, which changes all the time. Indeed, it is difficult to capture even when there are price signals, as Marks & Spencer, IBM, Dunlop and others have shown in failing to gather, comprehend, codify and respond swiftly to changes.

11 Karl Popper, *The Open Society and its Enemies* (London, Routledge & Kegan Paul, 1945); Robert Nozick, *Anarchy, State, and Utopia* (Oxford, Blackwell, 1974).

12 R.G.Evans, M.L.Barer, R.Marmot, *Why are Some People Healthy and Others Not?* (New York, Aldine de Gruyter, 1994)

13 Department of Health, *Working for Patients* (London, HMSO, 1989; Department of Health, *The Patient's Charter* (London, HMSO, 1991); White Paper, *The Citizen's Charter. Raising The Standard* (London, HMSO, 1991); *Citizen's Charter. First Report* 1992 (London, HMSO, 1992); NHS Executive, *Local Voices, The Views of Local People in Purchasing for Health* (London, Department of Health, 1992; *NHS Patient Partnership Strategy* (1996); Secretary of State for Health, *The New NHS. Modern, Dependable* (London, Department of Health, 1997), and Secretary of State for Health, *The NHS Plan: a Plan for Investment, a Plan for Reform* (London, Stationery Office, 2000). Also, Julian Le Grand et al, *Learning from the NHS Internal Market. A Review of the Evidence* (London, King's Fund, 1998), and W.Anderson and D.Florin, *One of Many Priorities. Public Involvement in Primary Care Groups* (London, King's Fund, 2000). The emphasis on the politicised activist user has had little real value in terms of local democracy, either. See S.Gillam and F.Brooks, *New Beginnings. Toward Patient and Public Involvement in Primary Care* (London, King's Fund, 2001). Also, Leigh Richardson, *Promoting Patient Participation in Portsmouth.* MBA Consultancy Project. Ashridge, Herts., Ashridge Management College, 1997.

14 Ben Russell, 'Trouble-shooters to be sent into ailing hospitals,' the *Independent*, 12 February 2002. Second leader, 'A small reform that points to a much bigger failure', the *Independent*, 12 February 2002. Senior managers were replaced at Ashford, Chertsey, Dartford & Gravesham, and Chase Farm, North London. But another six zero-rated Trusts were said to have made 'significant improvements' and avoided censure. No data was published by which this judgement could be assessed independently.

15 Will Anderson and Steve Gillam, 'The elusive NHS consumer: 1948 to the NHS Plan,' *Economic Affairs*, Vol.21, No.4, December 2001, pp.14-18.

16 Simon Jenkins, ''What the Tories need are some local heroes,' *The Times*, 18 January 2002, and his *Accountable to None: The Tory Nationalisation of Britain* (London, Hamish Hamilton, 1995). For a picture of what might happen if the local government route is followed, combined with much more health activism, see Rosie Ilett and Sue Laughlin, 'Devolving health and building a healthy Scotland. From the medical to the social model in the post-devolution environment', *Renewal*, Vol.9. No.1, Winter 2001, pp.26–35.

17 Milton Friedman, *Capitalism and Freedom* (Chicago, Chicago University Press, 1962); Milton & Rose Friedman, *Free To Choose, A Personal Statement* (New York, Harcourt Brace, 1980).

18 James M.Buchanan and Gordon Tullock, *The Calculus of Consent* (Ann Arbor, Michigan, University of Michigan Press, 1962); J.M.Buchanan, *The Limits of Liberty. Between Anarchy and Leviathan* (Chicago, Chicago University Press, 1975); Gordon Tullock, *The Vote Motive* (London, IEA, 1976); Arthur Seldon, *Capitalism* (Oxford, Blackwell, 1990).

19 Celia Hall, 'Heart surgery death leagues bring new fears for patients', *Daily Telegraph*, 18 January 2002.

20 T.McKeown, *The Role of Medicine: Dream, Mirage or Nemesis?* (Oxford, Blackwell, 1979); R.E.G.Evans, 'The dog in the night-time: medical practice variations and health policy', in T.V.Anderson and G.Mooney (eds.), *The Challenges of Medical Practice Variation*, Economic Issues in Health care Series (London, Macmillan Press, 1990); J.B.McKinley and S.M.McKinley, 'The questionable contribution of medical measures to the decline of mortality in the United States in the twentieth century', *Milbank Memorial Fund Quarterly, Health and Society*, Vol..55, No.3, 1977; R.G.Evans, M.L.Barer, R.Marmot, *Why are Some People Healthy and Others Not?* (New York, Aldine de Gruyter, 1994);, D.S.Lees, *Health Through Choice. An Economic Study of the British National Service* (London, Institute of Economic Affairs, 1961; Heinz Redwood, *Why Ration Health care? An international study of the United Kingdom, France, Germany and public sector health care in the USA* (London, Civitas, 2000);. Rosie Ilett and Sue Laughlin, 'Devolving health and building a healthy Scotland. From the medical to the social model in the post-devolution environment', *Renewal*, Vol.9. No.1, Winter 2001, pp.26-35; see also R. Ilett and K.Munro, 'Introducing the social model of health', in P.Craig and G.Lindsay (eds.), 2000, *Nursing and Public Health* (London, Harcourt Publishers, 2000).

21 D.S.Lees, *Health Through Choice. An Economic Study of the British National Service* (London, Institute of Economic Affairs, 1961). I owe this reference to Lord Ralph Harris.

The Watford gap

a view from the doorstep

Michael McManus

The Watford Constituency – consisting of the area covered by Watford Borough Council, plus smallish areas to the north and south – could almost be described as 'England writ small'. Within its confines are to be found all the aspirations, problems and challenges that typify the people of this country. With regard to the public services, the challenges and problems are much the same as those to be found in London – which begins on the boundaries of the constituency. As the candidate in Watford – a target seat – I felt myself to be in a different universe from those at Westminster who traded ideological statements and statistics.

Day after day I would be confronted with the shortcomings of the police service, our transport infrastructure, the secondary transfer system – and the National Health Service. Day after day I was also profoundly impressed by the dedication of the professionals involved in providing those services.

There are those who say that there is no such thing as a 'public service ethos'. They are wrong. Too often, however, those fine and idealistic intentions can be submerged under the weight of an inappropriate system imposed from above. As any candidate ought to appreciate (though one would hardly guess it from listening to the media) the NHS and its related services do not consist exclusively of doctors and nurses who work in hospitals. This is a huge and complicated system, embracing everything from home helps to rehabilitation centres and, at least according to some definitions, nursing and care homes.

The public services in a place like Watford suffer from the cost of living and, in particular, the high cost of housing. Recruitment and retention are extremely difficult in a setting where the cost of living is just as high as that in London, while at best only a reduced London weighting is available to staff. At every level within the service, this makes it difficult to attract people of high calibre. We have to depend on their willingness to make sacrifices. Fortunately, many of them do. According to the accounts of patients and the evidence of my own eyes, the state of the NHS in the town matches a familiar pattern.

Watford's general practitioners are a fairly go-getting bunch (they are, let it always be remembered, a fully 'privatised' part of the service), busily improving services and building extensions to their premises. There is more day surgery taking place in their practices all the time and they continue to make the most of the fact that they still enjoy at least some of the freedoms and powers that they gained under the last Conservative government.

They have their frustrations of course: like everyone else in the public services, they complain that their professional lives are blighted by arbitrary targets set from on high, and they find that 'reformed' budgeting arrangements create odd incentives for them. On the whole, however, they remain the most admired part of the NHS. The social services locally are more of a mixed bag, sometimes excellent and sometimes stretched to the limit, but it is at the General Hospital where the worst problems are to be found. It is based in some pretty run-down buildings next-door to a First Division football ground, in a traffic blackspot. It has problems filling vacancies, from the highest consultant to the humblest cleaner. Once again, the cost of living plays its part in that. The main problem, however, has nothing specifically to do with the medical staff, for Watford General Hospital was on the list of hospitals 'named and shamed' by the Government in the run-up to the general election as one of the dirtiest in the United Kingdom. I myself had heard so many horror stories of blood on sheets, curtains or floors that this particular announcement told me nothing new. Although few local people can have been surprised, this still came as a blow to prestige of the town.

The other main problem that I kept encountering was another one only too familiar to most of those who are engaged either in politics or in the NHS itself. In too many instances the NHS is still anything but a 'joined up' service. Too many people are leaving hospital too early, often to return in urgent need of further treatment. All too often the connections between health and personal social services are overstretched and inadequate. Too many people are returning from hospital to a home that is unheated, or empty, or simply ill-equipped for a convalescent person. I found the reaction to all of this on the doorstep most instructive. Certainly there was a sense – fairly or unfairly – that the Labour Party probably had a stronger commitment to the NHS than the Tories did, a sense echoed by the data in Andrew Cooper's essay. There was also a sense that we had spent too little on the NHS, that Labour was indeed trying to make up for our 'neglect' of the NHS. But there was another aspect that I found far more surprising. By and large, people suddenly seemed to have come to the view that it wasn't 'all about money'. They increasingly recognise that, in a vast institution such as the NHS, effective organisation is terribly important. Unless and until they were convinced that their hard-earned money was going straight through to the frontline, they were not at all keen to pay more taxes for the Health Service, nor indeed for any public service. I have since discovered that opinion polls since 2001 have detected a similar, marked shift in people's views towards the NHS. Once again Watford seemed to speak for the nation.

In a way, this was a victory for common sense, for it is plainly the case that the problems of the NHS will not be solved purely and simply by throwing more money at them. Nonetheless, by most standards the NHS is actually rather efficient. Furthermore, people do still like it and, so far as one could make out on the frontline, they adhered to its founding principle, namely that (in the words of the 1945 Conservative Party manifesto) 'the health services of the country will be made available to all citizens …

Everyone will contribute to the cost, and no one will be denied the attention, the treatment or the appliances he requires because he cannot afford them'. I would never care to stand for an election in the interest of a party that wished to depart from those basic principles. However, I did come to feel that there are quite radical changes that we could consider as a party without alienating the mainstream of public opinion, and without crossing the Rubicon by abandoning support for a universal service.

The health debate has moved on apace since the general election, largely as a consequence of the work done on behalf of Gordon Brown, under the chairmanship of Derek Wanless, looking into the long-term options for the NHS. In March last year, the Chancellor asked Mr Wanless to 'examine the technological, demographic and medical trends over the next two decades that may affect the health service in the UK as a whole'. The terms of reference left the door open for either extending charges within the NHS on a crudely means-tested basis (as in the case of eye or dental tests and prescriptions), or moving towards an element of hypothecation. There is no mention of services being 'free at the point of delivery' or even 'largely free at the point of delivery' – just a commitment (presumably unconsciously) echoing that Conservative one from 1945 – to a 'publicly funded, comprehensive, high quality service available on the basis of clinical need and not ability to pay'. Mr Wanless and his team were not asked to consider the question of how the NHS is – or should be – financed. They have already gone beyond their remit, therefore, with a statement in their interim report (published in November) that 'the current UK system for financing health care shapes up well against the alternatives'. Gordon Brown seized upon this at once, appearing to claim that the debate about how the NHS should be financed was now effectively at an end.

In fact, most of the evidence presented in the interim Wanless Report suggests that something is very badly wrong with the NHS. Survival rates for cancer and heart patients are well below where they should be. Life expectancy, especially for women, is below where it might be. We have fewer doctors and nurses per head than we should. The most striking figure, however, is for the amount that we spend on healthcare here in the UK. Despite the commitment to the NHS of successive governments since 1948, the latest figures suggest that we spend a lower proportion of national income on healthcare than any similar country does. In 1998 we spent 6.8 per cent of GDP on healthcare – compared with 8.7 per cent in Holland, 9.3 per cent in France and Canada, and 10.3 per cent in Germany. The proportion of national income spent on public healthcare here is even lower than the figure for the USA, where so much more private money is spent.

Having spent the first two months of 2002 working on a healthcare research project, I know only too well that many aspects of this debate are as old as the NHS, or even older. Perhaps what struck me most forcibly was my discovery that every government since 1948 has come into office pledging to decentralise within the NHS, to give more power to doctors and other healthcare professionals. Yet there has been precious little achieved in that direction, with the possible exception of the Clarke reforms of the late 1980s. The present government, with its bizarre love of targets and tables for everything, has done more damage than most. These targets have generally distorted more than they have helped. Statements by ministers are always high on grandeur, absurdly *de haut en bas*, rarely resonating with those – either patients or professionals – on the frontline. There has also been a reluctance, for all the cant about 'reform', to recognise that lessons can be learned from practice elsewhere – notably Europe, but also from that other 'foreign country' the past. I am sure that the Conservative Party was right to risk evoking images of Hattie Jacques and Kenneth Williams with its call last year for the return of matrons to our hospitals. Bureaucrats at the top of a hospital are all very well, but it is more often down at ward level where an absence of effective management is so very obvious.

The great argument between Labour and Conservative during the debates that led to the foundation of the NHS in 1948 centred on the future of the voluntary hospitals. Most Tories strongly supported the creation of a National Health Service, but they felt that the old voluntary hospitals should be allowed to tie up with local government rather than central government. The Labour view, inimitably embodied by Aneurin Bevan, was that there should be nothing less than a nationalisation of healthcare – a 'takeover', no less. This led to the notorious Second Reading debate in the House of Commons, during which one Conservative after another spoke up in favour of the new NHS, whereupon the party voted *en masse* against it. Decentralisation has a surprisingly strong resonance with the electorate. They have seen for themselves that the 'big is always better' school has got it wrong on health, and they want to sense that we are now serious about giving medical professionals – and local people more generally – a greater say in local healthcare.

Another issue that really concerns people is the question of residential care for the elderly. Many are aware of what has now happened in Scotland, and there is a great deal of support for a similar shift in England. Whenever I spoke to anyone involved in the running of a care home, I found them to be at their wits' end. They are caught between the Scylla of rising property prices and the Charybdis of a bureaucratic and inefficient system for getting paid. In an increasing number of instances, it just isn't worth running a care home anymore. The knock-on effects for the NHS, and hospitals in particular, are disastrous. It is also high time that, without compromising their independence from the state, we looked at ways of helping the hospices more. They are so often the unsung heroes of the healthcare system, yet we do so take them for granted.

If we are to do more, how are we to pay for it? I think we do have to take serious note of the increasing scepticism of many taxpayers towards the notion that more money is the answer to everyone's woes. I have no doubt that people are willing to put their hands in their pockets for healthcare – if, and only if, they are convinced that the money is going to have a direct effect on the quality of frontline services. There are two basic ways of linking what people pay more closely with what they get. I would not fancy selling the idea of extended charging on the doorstep. People need to believe that we share their belief in the principles of the NHS. The more noises we make about charging, the more we sow doubts in their minds. I'm also convinced that it's not much good saying that payments will be 'means-tested'. This usually means that the costs of a service continue to fall disproportionately on those whose incomes put them on just the wrong side of some arbitrary line. When we defend the existing charges, we can be rather too glib in saying that they only have to be paid by 'those who can afford them'. Well, some people can afford them a lot more easily than others and I think we must be careful about creating new complications in the benefits and taxation system – or new poverty traps.

A lot of our health policy at the 2001 general election was rather good, and stood up to the rigours of an election campaign. It is surely right that people who are waiting care not one jot for the length of the queue – they are understandably more concerned about how long they will have to wait. Our criticisms of the 'postcode lottery' also struck home, though I am not sure that we yet have an answer on that one, given that resources are inevitably finite and demands infinite. After all the meetings and speeches and seminars and doorstep interrogations I also do now think we should have a long, hard look at various forms of tax hypothecation for healthcare, perhaps through the national insurance system, and at new ways of decentralising healthcare and recreating at least some of the spirit of the old voluntary hospitals that achieved so much before 1948. We are still a serious political party – serious about winning the arguments, and winning future elections – and that surely means that at every stage we should confine ourselves to policy options that are likely to commend themselves to mainstream public opinion. By and large people like their NHS, largely free at the point of delivery, and they are willing to pay for it. They also believe that it's the job of politicians to run it competantly for them. If we try to tell them that they are wrong in this, they in turn are surely perfectly entitled to conclude that we aren't worth voting for. We now owe it to ourselves, and to the country, to make ourselves electable again.

Beyond left and right

The challenge of a free market in healthcare

Dr Tim Evans Ph.D

In 1948, the government issued a leaflet to every home in Britain. Extolling the virtues of the new National Health Service (NHS) 'the NHS' it read 'will provide you with all medical, dental and nursing care. Everyone – rich or poor – can use it.'[1] The key word here was the word *all*. The state was going to fund comprehensive and universal healthcare for everyone.

Today, one cannot open a newspaper without reading about the pressures and strains on the NHS. Half a century on from its inception, the NHS is failing to make good its late 1940s promises. Beyond the world of political hype and media spin, rationing, through a number of means, has always been rife in the service and patients have often been denied the timely and high quality treatments that they perhaps could have otherwise had.

Today, higher expectations and new technology are fueling ever increasing demands on a health system which are impossible to meet via the old methods of top-down state control.

Yet, in attempting to get to grips with these problems, it is important for the Conservatives to acknowledge that the government has made some bold and necessary advances in recent years, changes which not only move health policy in the right direction but illuminate where it might travel further in the years to come.

After years of shunning liberal, market based, solutions in healthcare it is this Labour government that has introduced a concordat with the independent sector, whereby NHS-funded patients can receive treatment in independent hospitals. It is this government that is mobilising private hospitals on the continent for the benefit of NHS-patients. And it is Labour that is now planning to return NHS hospitals to the pre-1948 world of genuine independence from the state under the rubric of not-for-profit Foundation Hospitals.

Perhaps most importantly of all, it is this government which is overseeing a funding revolution in private health spending which, as yet, has not been fully explored by the Conservatives.

The concordat and beyond

The success of the concordat between the NHS and independent hospitals, whereby more than 100,000 NHS patients have received high quality NHS-funded treatment and care in independent hospitals, is a testimony to the pragmatism of this government.

Allowing NHS patients to use independent hospitals on the continent when local NHS or independent hospitals are unable to help also makes sense. Moreover, the recently announced policy of allowing the best NHS hospitals to become completely independent from the state as Foundation Hospitals is a departure from post-war Labour thinking without precedent.

State of independence

It was the Secretary of State for Health, Alan Milburn who recently asserted:

> For fifty years the NHS has been subject to day-to-day running from Whitehall. The whole system is top down. There is little freedom for local innovation or risk taking. . . . A million strong health service cannot be run from Whitehall. Indeed, it should not be run from Whitehall. For patient choice to thrive it needs a different environment. One in which there is greater diversity and plurality in local services which have the freedom to innovate and respond to patients needs. Our reforms are about redefining what we mean by the National Health Service. Changing it from a monolithic, centrally-run, monopoly provider of services to a values-based system where different health care providers – in the public, private and voluntary sectors – provide comprehensive services to NHS patients. . . . Who provides the service becomes less important than the service that is provided.[2]

Healthcare in Britain is changing, and the signs from the government are increasingly clear: the NHS is destined to become a regulator and a funder of health services, it will not necessarily be a provider or owner of facilities.

Sir Keith Joseph on New Labour

In the last article he wrote for the *Daily Telegraph* before he died in 1996, Sir Keith Joseph argued that market based institutions in civil society should be rediscovered and applied to health and welfare. Prophetically, he wrote:

> My own favorite strategy to give every home a stake in the economy is to allow Friendly Societies to recover much of the role they relinquished over this century. No pension fund, state or corporate, conveys a sense of ownership or participation. I believe the small mutual status of Friendly Societies keeps the quality of co-operative intimacy. [3]

Today, six years on from writing these wise words, it is Alan Milburn who has recently said:

> Last month, I met with the chief executives of the three star [NHS] Trusts. They had a list of further specific restrictions that they wanted to have removed from them and we are now considering how best to do so. But they also asked us to go further. If they were as good as we agreed they were, why could they not become independent not-for-profit institutions with just an annual cash for performance contract and no further form of performance management from the centre?[4]

In outlining the government's ideas for genuinely independent 'Foundation Hospitals' the Secretary of State continued:

> This middle ground between state-run public and shareholder-led private structures is where there has been growing interest in recent years. Both the Right – through organisations like the Institute of Directors – and the Left – through the Co-operative Movement – have been examining the

> case for new forms of organisation such as mutuals or public interest companies . . .'[5]

Keith Joseph had warned of such politics coming from New Labour back in 1996. He well understood that the race to capture such terrain was on between the two major parties. He wrote in his *Daily Telegraph* article:

> I wonder if the Labour Party hungry for radical ideas, might steal such notions and apply them first. I regard Frank Field MP as our most dangerous opponent as he treats liberal market ideas as serious options, and not merely as misanthropy. [6]

Mapping out the radical and strategic aim of returning NHS hospitals to the world of independence, Alan Milburn concluded his speech in early 2002 by saying of Foundation Hospitals:

> Some will see this as a very controversial step . . . And it is worth putting into a slightly broader context. No other country in Europe, including those with a strong centre left tradition, would blink an eyelid at these plans. At the time the NHS was being formed as a nationalised industry in the UK, elsewhere in Europe many socialist or social democrat governments forged institutions which favored greater community ownership over state ownership. Even here there is a long and honourable tradition within the British Labour movement of developing local community and self-help organisations.'[7]

Capturing traditionally Conservative and classical liberal terrain in one fell swoop, Milburn concluded:

> In many other European countries there are many not-for-profit voluntary or charity-run hospitals all providing care to the public health care system. There are private sector organisations doing the same. Similar steps are already starting here. We are in negotiations with BUPA…[8]

The unintended consequences of health nationalisation

In its historic form, the NHS has always presented its political masters with the same challenge. Namely, that of managing a service which is based – in the public's mind at least – on the promise of providing unlimited healthcare free and available at the point of delivery.

In reality, it did not take the 1945 Labour government long to realize that the NHS was not going to keep up with – or reduce as some had suggested – people's demand for healthcare.[9] While a number of experts had popularised the view that there might be an 'initial surge' in demand for spectacles and false teeth and then demand would decrease, it soon became clear that such theorising was nonsense.

Back in 1944, the government WhitePaper, *A National Health Service*, estimated that the service would cost taxpayers £132 million per year. However, this was revised upwards to £152 million in 1946 and again to £230 million just before the Act came into force in July 1948. In its first full year of operation –

1949–50 – the NHS actually ended up costing £305 million and required a supplementary estimate of £98 million.[10]

The early estimates of expenditure were ultimately inaccurate because the government not only assumed that the service would account for a small and stable share of public expenditure but because their projections were based on extrapolations of pre-war spending levels which were mainly on cheaper preventative measures.

The inaccuracy of the estimates can be attributed to a number of factors. The first was that the early projections of cost assumed that demand would remain roughly constant, despite there being no price constraints on demand – the service being 'free' at the point of use.

Secondly, contemporary social and medical developments exacerbated the problems created by an absence of any price constraints on demand, not least because medical advances at the time meant that there was a dramatic expansion in the type and range of health services which could be made available.

Again, the NHS was designed in many ways to provide a style of health care that was more appropriate to the 19th century rather than the 20th. Previous improvements in health had been brought about through large scale immunisation and better sanitation and nutrition. These measures had been relatively inexpensive, easy to administer and subject to large economies of scale.

The 20th century, however, characteristically saw the development of treatments for a range of degenerative conditions and most of these have tended to require a range of costly individual actions and medications. Crucially, effective treatments for degenerative conditions have not lowered health costs in the way that the eradication of conditions like smallpox once did.

Importantly, the number of people most likely to suffer these degenerative conditions has steadily increased as life expectancy rates have improved, placing further pressures on healthcare. In 1901, for example, people over the age of 50 comprised just 14.8 per cent of the United Kingdom's population, whereas by 1951 they accounted for 27.6 per cent. By 1981 the figure had reached 31.8 per cent and continues to rise.[11]

The government realised early on that it could not afford a health service that was entirely free at the point of use. Although this was one of the founding principles of the NHS, it was actually abandoned within five years of the 1944 White Paper. In 1949, an amending Act was passed to allow the levying of a one shilling charge on prescriptions. After the Conservative election victory of 1951, further charges were introduced for prescriptions, spectacles and dental treatment. Indeed, it was as far back as 1956 that the present scheme of levying prescription charges by the number of items prescribed was first introduced.

The aim of these charging mechanisms was to simultaneously open a new source of funding revenue for the NHS whilst also deterring 'frivolous' demand for healthcare. But these measures proved to be grossly inadequate. For while there was some slowing in the rate of increase in the prescriptions issued, the revenue raised was never as significant as the Treasury would have liked. In 1950–51, charges contributed less than one per cent to the NHS budget and even their largest contribution later in the decade was only 5.3 per cent.[12]

Another check on demand was a more deliberate rationing of supply – through scarcity rather than price. While doctors who worked in NHS hospitals had been encouraged at first to treat their patients according to need and not to be deterred by financial considerations, the imposition of cash limits soon turned them into allocators of scarce resources.

More than minimal care was denied to cases where there was little chance of successful recovery, particularly to young children or the elderly with serious conditions. Indeed, healthcare for everyone else was provided sparingly by international standards. In the late 1970s for example coronary artery by-pass operations were performed about ten times more frequently in America than in Britain. And where these did not increase life expectancy, they tended to reduce adverse symptoms such as pain. While American doctors responded to complaints about pain, British doctors have tended to pay more attention to the probable increases in life expectancy, or the improvements in a 'quality of life' not always synonymous with an absence of serious discomfort.[13]

The supply of healthcare has again been rationed still further by queuing. Crowded waiting rooms are common in most general practices and out-patient departments. And queues have become a fact of life for in-patients, often with long waiting periods for those operations given priority. Even in the 1980s and 1990s, after years of reforms designed to cut waiting lists, the median time to have a hernia repaired was more than 10 weeks and 14 for having a cataract treated.[14] The waiting times for many other less urgent procedures have usually been measured in months.

Certain health services have never been provided by the NHS, reducing the demand on its resources still further. Most forms of cosmetic surgery have rarely been available and face lifts, liposuction, hair transplants and sex change operations have never been provided except where they have been deemed necessary for reasons of health or as part of some other form of treatment. Other services have been provided on a minimal basis too. Much psychiatry, the treatment of infertility and substance misuse services are cases in point.

Against the popular view that the NHS exists to provide 'free' and virtually unlimited healthcare, history demonstrates that the supply of NHS services has always been limited in significant ways. In reality, people have never had an absolute right to free and equal treatment on demand in the NHS. What they have had, in the main, is an unlimited right of access to a waiting list from which, with a few exceptions, they will not be excluded. This right of access is not equivalent to a right to treatment, as any notional right to treatment has little value in practice if it is only available at the end of a two year waiting time. The right to healthcare is unlimited in the long term, but is strictly limited in the short term when healthcare is actually required to relieve pain or discomfort at the very least.

Significantly for the future of the UK's health and welfare

debate, rationing will continue to increase in importance because the demands placed upon the NHS will continue to expand. There are many fundamental demographic, technological, surgical and pharmaceutical developments that are, over time, continuing to increase the cost of healthcare and hence the demands placed upon the service. Cultural changes will also continue to have a major impact. As patients' expectations are raised alongside higher living standards so ever larger numbers of people are finding the unresponsive nature of state healthcare unacceptable.

It is in this context that it can be expected that an ever larger number of people will continue to return to the more sustainable tradition of voluntary self-help and the free market. As people become accustomed to improvements in customer service in other areas of life so the NHS is finding it increasingly difficult to run the risk of being exposed as an unacceptably customer unfriendly organisation.

Funding issues

At present, Labour claims that it is only the Conservatives who want to encourage various forms of private health funding. Yet today, under Labour's governance, seven million people have private medical insurance and another seven million people are covered by private health cash plans. Millions more choose from a wide range of other private funding options.

In the year 2000, more than a quarter of a million people chose to self-fund for independent acute hospital surgery and treatment without any insurance at all. Instead, they simply paid cash or via their credit cards. In dentistry, more than a third of the population has now abandoned the NHS and relies solely on independent sector treatment. And more than eight million people pay privately for a range of complimentary medical therapies every year.

According to recent research published in the *Daily Telegraph*[15], more than 3.5 million trade unionists – over 50 per cent of the Trade Union Congress's 6.8 million members – now enjoy the benefits of private health cash and medical insurance schemes. As reported, supporters of the movement even have their own web site at www.tradeunion-privatehealth.org.uk.

The future is independent

Just as the Labour Party shunned independent healthcare providers only a few years ago, so it is important for the Conservatives to ask how Tony Blair might want to play this important trade union card Under pressure for more reform, might the Prime Minister use this element of his own movement to help create a 'Stakeholder Health Funding' mechanism for the low-paid in the future and thereby attempt to outmaneuvrer the centre-right?[16] In a world beyond independent sector partnerships in provision and Foundation Hospitals might the Prime Minister want to take Sir Keith Joseph's ideas a stage further in health funding and capture still more Conservative terrain? Perhaps only time will tell.

At a time when the whole political class is trying to get itself off the hook for past political promises concerning the NHS, it is important that the Conservatives understand that many independent sector organisations already have established links with trade unions or have large numbers of trade unionists in membership. It is important that they think through the policy implications of such arrangements and who might seek to capture this political terrain in the not too distant future.

Some schemes offer private medical, permanent health or critical illness cover. Others offer private health cash benefits that pay for services which include items such as dentistry, ophthalmics, physiotherapy, chiropody, podiatry, maternity services, allergy testing, hospital in-patient stays, nursing home stays, hospital day case admissions, convalescence, home help, mental health and psychiatric treatment and, in some cases, even the use of an ambulance.

Today, independent sector not-for-profit organisations such as the Benenden Hospital, Bristol Contributory Welfare Association, BUPA, Civil Service Healthcare Society, Hospital Savings Association, Simplyhealth, Standard Life Healthcare, Wakefield Health Scheme, Westfield Contributory Health Scheme and dozens of other similar bodies, have millions of trade unionists in their combined memberships.[17]

Many public sector trade unions such as Unison even have formal links with private health cash schemes such as Medicash and promote them on their internet sites. These schemes are an important and growing source of revenue for the independent sector and add to the diversity of the overall health market.

The new politics of health

In reality, the old NHS is already dead. The idea of the state owning all health facilities and providing all services free at the point of delivery was always a utopian fantasy destined to fail.

Having been born of an independent sector estate that was founded with the establishment of St Bartholomew's Hospital in 1123, British healthcare is once again returning to a rich and diverse tapestry of independent sector provision and funding for its future.

With private expenditure on healthcare and insurance growing, and ever larger numbers of trade unionists turning to private health schemes rooted in civil society, it is clear that healthcare is slowly going back to the future. When it comes to the politics of modern healthcare and the radicalism presented by New Labour, Sir Keith Joseph's libertarian vision must remain the Conservative's guide. For it is in the context of his free market ideas that politicians of all parties find themselves today mere corks bobbing on the tide of history. A tide upon which politicians are firmly identified as being the problem and not the solution in people's healthcare.

1 Department of Health leaflet, July 1948.

2 The Secretary of State for Health, the Rt. Hon. Alan Milburn MP, speech to New Health Network, 15 January 2002.

3 Sir Keith Joseph, Why the Tories are the real party of the stakeholder, *Daily Telegraph*, 12 January 1996.

4 Alan Milburn, op. cit.

5 Ibid.

6 Keith Joseph, op. cit.

7 Alan Milburn, op. cit.

8 Ibid.

9 Rudolf Klein, *The Politics of the National Health Service*, Longman, London, 2nd edition, 1989, p.35.

10 Ibid., p.34.

11 David and Gareth Butler, *British Political Facts 1900–1985,* Macmillan Press, Basingstoke, 6th edition, 1986, p.235.

12 Klein, op.cit., p.39.

13 Henry J Aron and William R. Schwartz, *The Painful Prescription: Rationing Hospital Care,* Brookings Institute, Washington DC, 1984, p.67.

14 Klein, op.cit., p.155.

15 Daniel Kruger, 'Why half the members of trade unions have private health care', *Daily Telegraph*, 11 September 2001.

16 For a leading libertarian-Conservative academic who has long argued that Blair's inner coterie is planning such a move see: Nigel Ashford, (1997) New Labour's Hidden Agenda: Tony Blair's Plan to Privatise Health and Welfare, *Political Notes* No.136, Libertarian Alliance, London. This paper is available online at www.libertarian.co.uk

17 For more information on the involvement of trade union leaders in independent healthcare see: How union chiefs joined a private health plan, *Daily Mail,* 3 September 2001; Union bosses had health cover, the *Sunday Times*, 2 September 2001.

A private view

Mark Bassett

Introduction

Fifteen years ago I read a book that changed my life; *National Health* by John Vaizey, the father of the editor of this publication.

From that day, health services management has been my consuming passion. It has taken me all over the western world, from San Francisco to Svedlovsk, from Quarry House to BUPA House, and from a gay and lesbian project in Greenwich Village NY to the Presidential Palace in Warsaw. It's been an absorbing journey, and one that has enabled me to observe the dynamics of various health systems in diverse roles and from different perspectives.

The invitation to contribute to this book prompted me to re-read *National Health*. Having done that I intend to use this chapter for four purposes: to review what Lord Vaizey wrote, to summarize some of what has happened to the UK health system in the intervening years, to suggest a direction for the further reform of the UK health system and finally to offer some thoughts on the wider implications of that suggestion. The chapter reflects my personal views and thus represents a private view in both senses of the word. It's also a fiercely non-party political view. In both my professional and private lives I am happy to work with all parties, but aim to be beholden to none.

National Health

National Health is an unusual book. Its analysis and diagnosis was entirely unconventional, its proposed treatment radical, but subtle and sensitive. It is a polemic, yet balanced and thoughtful. I believe it remains a model of its kind. But what of its content?

Lord Vaizey's main thesis was that treatable illnesses are growing and changing fast. Good health services, he asserted, need to be able to respond quickly by changing in manner and location. Modern health care is concerned with the organisation of a system to meet changing patterns of demand. He highlighted increasing tension between the counselling, caring and curing functions of the medical profession. He argued for a change of emphasis between hospital and primary care and for an increased emphasis on 'preventive health care'. More broadly he argued firmly that health policy should be better aligned with wider social and economic policy. 'Medicine is marginal (though crucial) to the main problem – the question of the way of life of the community.'

His views on the organisational problems of the NHS were very specific: 'At the moment the hospital is organised around the consultant and his or her facilities. An 800-bed hospital may well employ more than 5,000 people. It is this concentration of people that, in the absence of good management, tax management skills, leads to poor productivity, high costs and demotivation. If only productivity could be raised, efficiency would rise as well'. High technology, he argued, has changed the emphasis and intensity of health care. Hospitals deal with the more serious cases, but with decreasing numbers of patients in bed. The urgent need, he said, is to make hospitals more efficient and divert resources to primary care.

Vaizey justified and proposed his principal solution to these problems very succinctly: 'the changing pattern of demand creates different problems of supply from those caused by a simple fall or rise in demand in an existing pattern of supply... The thesis of this book is that the organisation (of health services) should be diverse and decentralised and that financial sources should be widened to include state, insurance and personal spending'.

From an economic perspective Vaizey also asserted that 'Health care is not a drain on output if people need it and are prepared to pay for it' and that 'rising expenditure is not synonymous with rising costs. Rising expenditure is desirable if it gives people what they want – more comfortable, happier lives with less ill health.'

In his final chapters Vaizey returns to justify further and amplify his main themes with some policy proposals and guidelines:

- The wider definition of health care and the rising wealth of the community demand a diversity of provision.
- It is highly likely (and desirable) that this will entail a diversity of sources of funding.
- The vital matter is to encourage freedom to experiment and innovate and to reward success. Attempts to control priorities and to limit profit is certain to be shortsighted and to slow down medical progress.

- Differences of payment and provision seem to have surprisingly little effect on outcomes, mortality or morbidity rates, or the take-up of medical care. But they deeply affect the style of provision, the attitudes of the public and the remuneration of doctors.
- A central part of modern medical practice, therefore, is not only adequate record keeping, but also access to records kept by others, notably the hospital, the school and the social services ... it is essential that all relevant information be available to the medical practitioner, whether he is in private practice or public service.
- There is no administrative reason why patients should not 'top-up' the state system of finance with contribution of private fees, plus whatever private insurance might provide.
- Uniformity is not compatible with medical progress ... the pressure for uniformity arises from a misplaced notion that medical care is 'urgent and essential'. Some is, most of it is not.
- Social services for the elderly and mentally ill should be linked to the primary health care team.
- The development of modern communication techniques should make ... communication far simpler. Computerised hospital records ought to be mutually compatible with general practice records, which in turn, should be linked to pharmacies and other para-medical records.
- NHS administration exists predominantly to control costs and allocate resources. By far the simplest way to do this is for the funding agency to pay unit per item of service... There is no reason why the standard cost per item should not be paid to private hospitals and clinics.
- It would be essential to challenge the idea of national scales of salaries and wages.

Lord Vaizey concluded by defining the key responsibilities of Government in the system he advocated: to determine the desired level of public expenditure, to allocate resources and to ensure that the money allocated was spent effectively. Vaizey asserts 'what individuals spend in excess of this – whether directly, or indirectly through insurance – should be their affair'.

The intervening years

I think that much has been achieved in the past fifteen years, by both Conservative and Labour Governments.

Many of these changes can be regarded as essential preliminaries to the more radical reform Vaizey envisaged. For example between 1985 and 1997 the Conservatives:

- Introduced the 'purchaser/provider split' into the NHS making the roles and responsibilities of 'commissioners' and 'providers' clearer.
- Introduced capital and total cost accounting into the NHS enabling both the ongoing assessment of the value of capital and enabling the NHS to purchase for 'best value' outside NHS organisations.
- Commenced primary care commissioning in the form of 'GP fundholding'. Over time this should help facilitate decision making between GP and patient about treatment and care and make the health system less hospital focused.
- Committed the Department of Health to the World Health Organisation Health For All approach to policy analysis and development. Over time this should help promote thinking about health policy as well as 'illness policy'.
- Introduced clinical audit on a voluntary basis.

- Re-organized specialist hospital services in London and concentrated resources and expertise in these expensive services into a more effective pattern of provision.

New Labour has also made many constructive steps forward since 1997 including:

- Radical improvements to the NHS system of performance management, giving increased emphasis on the potential effectiveness and efficiency of new technologies.
- Beginning to re-appraise and expand medical and nursing manpower planning, training and education.
- The extension of primary care commissioning throughout England through the creation of Primary Care Groups and Trusts.
- A major programme for the building and refurbishment of primary care facilities through NHS LIFT.
- Signing a Concordat with the independent healthcare sector to use private hospitals to provide NHS services when this represents best value.
- Legislating to integrate public social care entitlements with additional voluntary expenditure.

Last year the Chancellor also commissioned Derek Wanless to appraise future health trends and the financial and other resources that will be required by the NHS in 2020.

Lord Vaizey would have been delighted that the Chancellor is looking that far ahead but disappointed that Mr Wanless has no formal mandate to consider the contribution and resource implications of other organizations in the wider UK health and care system.

Lord Vaizey would also have been disappointed that, despite embarking on a major programme of hospital building, the Government has given no detailed consideration to the nature of hospital buildings needed in the coming years.

Whatever next?

Much has been done over the past fifteen years to identify and address deficiencies in the NHS. Strategy, structure, systems, skills, style, staff and 'shared values' have all been scrutinized. Many of the issues identified are still being rectified. Will addressing them be enough? Like Vaizey I think not.

The Government's underlying aim in health policy remains egalitarian; but people are in aims, attitudes and abilities all unique.

I believe that the Government would do better to if it sought to define concerted standards for UK residents in key policy areas such a housing, education, health, travel, recreation and employment. When these standards are met the rest, as Vaizey suggested, should be 'entirely our own affair'.

What issues arise? An important one is this – how to manage the relationship between such 'standards' or social protections for all and additional voluntary expenditure.

Let me use a relatively simple example. Train travel. Imagine that in ten years time the Government of the day decided to 'give' transport passes to everyone over sixty, the policy intentions being to promote travel by the elderly but at the same time to minimize traffic congestion and road traffic accidents involving elderly people.

If an older person wanted to upgrade to first class should they pay the full first class fare, or the difference between first and second class fare? I suggest that the latter is economically the most rational approach. The former would constrain demand forcing elderly people to pay 'full cost' for 'a marginal benefit'.

Over time any attempt to force the former position would erode demand amongst the elderly for first class rail travel. Would that improve the lot of elderly people who wanted to rely soley on their passes? No. It would rather harm their interests by reducing overall investment in locomotives and railtrack, when the elderly people who would otherwise have traveled by first class rail switch to private transport.

My inference is clear. Statute prohibits most approaches to 'topping up' NHS entitlements. People increasingly forgo some of their public entitlements because these do not meet their needs in a timely and effective manner. Support for the underlying principles of the NHS is put under strain, unnecessarily.

A better direction is clear. Commit to decent standards for all and encourage more investment in healthcare by allowing people to 'top up' their public entitlements with discretionary spending to meet their individual wants and needs. This is, I believe, the way to re-create a health and care system in the UK that can again become and remain 'the envy of the world'!

Wider implications

I believe that the UK electorate recognizes that the new global economy is tending to amplify differences in earning potential based on knowledge and skill. That is threatening to many in the UK and they will be looking to Government to protect key elements of their standard of living; either through financial re-distribution and/or improved public services.

Notwithstanding that, I believe that there is an appetite in the electorate for the further re-defining the role of government, politics and public services in the UK. As we enter the twenty first century all the major political parties have everything to play for if they, too, are to survive and thrive.

I went to an excellent talk by Howard Davies, the Director of the Financial Services Authority, recently. 'In the long run you will get the regulation you deserve' he remarked. The same I think is true in politics and public services. Change is rarely easy. John Vaizey set out why changing any health system is both necessary and particularly difficult. His book remains both relevant and readable. I hope we can complete the changes to our health and care system he envisaged during the coming fifteen years. It is technically possible. The key limiting factors are political, professional and managerial leadership. We will, then as now, have the system we deserve; nothing more, nothing less.

1 John Vaizey, *National Health* (Martin Robertson, 1984)

Public service not public sector

Combining social solidarity with consumer choice

David G. Green

The main problem the Conservatives face is the shallow and unscrupulous approach of Mr Blair. In January 2002 during his highly publicised Newcastle speech on the public services, he contrasted his preference for 'sustained investment matched with reform' to the rival view that 'the Thatcherite revolution was never completed and that the solution is to cut back on investment, cut taxes and then get people to purchase their own services'. If there were payment, he says, the top ten per cent may be able to afford it but 'the other 90 per cent will just be left with sink public services in a perpetual state of decline'. And 'let no one pretend', he thundered, that there is a choice between 'a public service which we pay for in taxes' and 'a private service that somehow comes free'.

Eh! Is he really making a contrast between a free private service and a public service you have to pay for? Let's hope that this risible comparison marks the lowest point to which the debate sinks.

The challenge for the Tories is to raise the tone of the debate by coming to terms with the plain facts that have escaped Mr Blair's attention. All health systems are paid for by the people who use them. We do not face a choice between payment and non-payment but between *methods* of payment – and some methods seem to work better than others. A good system of finance would address itself to three main concerns.

The first is how best to ensure we have got a system that allows the resources available for treatment at any moment to match current clinical need and consumer demand. Has the NHS method of payment from general taxation proved to be a good way to ensure that the number of doctors and hospitals, for instance, will be sufficient to meet established medical need? Or have other systems proved more effective? It has been accepted by many observers that the NHS has suffered from years of under-investment, but few have yet to acknowledge the reason, namely that there is no systematic connection between the tax revenues assigned to the NHS and medical need.

Second, looking around the world it is apparent that some methods of payment put service users in a weak position and some in a strong position. European social insurance systems empower their members to exercise a free choice of doctor. The French, for example, pay a social insurance premium calculated as a percentage of their income. They cannot vary this amount, but it entitles them to go to any doctor they want. The UK Treasury also takes money from our pay packets but, unlike in France, the result is to reduce our purchasing power and diminish our ability to choose.

Third, some methods encourage social solidarity between, on the one hand, the majority of the population who have gone out to work and earned enough to pay for the services they need and, on the other, the minority who cannot afford to pay. Mr Blair talks as if only 10 per cent of the population can afford to pay for healthcare. Who does he think is paying the taxes on which the NHS relies? In reality, the majority of us are net contributors to the public funds that finance the NHS.

What can we learn from social insurance schemes? Methods of paying for health care can be compared by asking three questions: about transparency, consumer control and social solidarity.

1 Can you tell how much you are paying, so that you are able to form a reasoned view about the value for money being offered?
2 What sort of control have you got over the agency that receives the money you pay?
3 Are the majority of middle-income earners able to ensure that the poorest members of society are receiving a good standard of care?

In another well-publicised speech, Mr Blair has said that people who sing the praises of the French system fail to distinguish between 'the impact of extra resources and the mechanism for raising the cash'. The interim Wanless report made a similar claim and concluded that there was little difference between tax and social insurance. Such claims, however, ignore the importance of making payments visible and neglect the empowering impact of paying an insurance premium to an organisation that represents the interests of consumers. Compare Germany, France, Switzerland and the UK.

In France people pay a percentage of their income, currently 7.5 per cent, and employers pay a percentage of payroll (12.8 per cent). This money goes to an independent agency which is run by a board comprising representatives of employers and employees. It empowers French people to choose the doctor or hospital they want.

In Germany, the cost is also expressed as a percentage of income and employers and employees pay half each. The average cost is 13.5 per cent of income. Again the money does not go to the German government, but to independent sickness funds which pay for the care chosen by their members. Germans are free to change funds.

In Switzerland, it is compulsory to pay for a basic insurance plan defined by law and about 100 non-profit private insurers compete for customers. Each company charges all its members the same premium, regardless of age. There are 23 cantons in Switzerland, each with a slightly different policy towards subsidisation. One approach is to cap the premium if it exceeds 10 per cent of taxable income; another is to pay on a sliding scale based on income. The very poor have the full premium paid for them so that everyone is an insured customer. People who want to pay for extras, over and above the basic plan can do so. But all have a stake in the standard package guaranteed for everyone. The Swiss system is particularly interesting because individuals pay personally for health insurance. Because there is no employer contribution, the Swiss have overcome one of the great difficulties of the German and French systems, namely that employers complain that they are unable to compete in global markets because of the high social costs they bear.

People who say that social insurance is just another tax are wrong. When we pay taxes in the UK the money goes to the Treasury which treats it as 'government money' not the consumer's. Under social insurance systems premiums are payments to third party insurers who are under a contractual obligation to serve customers.

Just as making our advance payment to the Treasury reduces our ability to influence the care we enjoy ourselves, so it also diminishes our capacity to influence the standard to be guaranteed for the poor. Social insurance systems, like those in France and Germany, have proved better able to secure the willing support of the majority of the population for a universally high standard. We should search for a mechanism that allows middle-income people to make a price-conscious choice about how much to spend on insuring themselves and then make their preference the measure of the standard of care to be guaranteed for the poor.

Despite Mr Blair's claim, all systems are paid for by people who have made themselves financially independent by going out to work. These same middle-income people must, in practice, pay both for their own care and that of the poor. This is the reality whatever the mix between taxation, social insurance and private insurance.

A step-by-step approach

So much for the lessons from overseas. But how can we make rapid progress to a higher standard of care when years of neglect have caused supply-side bottlenecks? A step-by-step approach to reform will be necessary.

Once the Blair reforms are implemented, there will be 28 strategic health authorities in England supervising a larger number of primary care trusts. The trusts are to be the main buyers of services from hospitals, which will be subject to a regime of inspections and monitoring by central government and semi-autonomous agencies. How could this system be made more responsive to consumers?

A 'core service' with supplementary insurance

If the NHS continued to be funded from taxes and provided a 'core service' it would be possible, as the interim Wanless report implied, to permit people to purchase supplementary insurance for extras, such as private rooms. This would allow additional funding to flow into mainstream hospitals and, over time, it might establish a new standard of care that would be politically difficult to withhold from everyone. The disadvantage of such a system is that in the short run it only benefits the most well-off sections of society. Other methods are available that would extend the benefits more widely.

Harnessing self-interest

The main challenge in the short run is to give middle-income people a good reason to pay a lot more for themselves and simultaneously to pay more for the poor. Whatever people say to opinion pollsters, they are not very likely to want to pay a lot more in taxes. However, a judicious combination of self-interest and social solidarity may have a better chance.

One approach would be to allow individuals to contract out of the NHS on condition that they take full personal responsibility for their own health care costs by purchasing an appropriate health insurance policy. They would still pay taxes and thus contribute to the NHS but, if they received a tax credit of about 50 per cent of the cost of their private insurance up to an agreed maximum, they would have a strong incentive to take responsibility for their own costs, thus adding to total health care resources as well as taking pressure off the NHS. In practice they would often have to use NHS hospitals for services, but they would be expected to pay and then reclaim from their insurer.

If confined only to those who could afford to buy a comprehensive insurance policy, it could lead to large additional investments which would also assist the least well off, albeit indirectly. However, once a fully functioning insurance market were established it would be possible to extend the freedom to contract out to everyone. In *Stakeholder Health Insurance* I discussed how this could be done to the advantage of all sections of society. It would involve setting up a consumer purchasing agency (a co-op) in each health authority. People who are satisfied need do nothing. Others may opt to receive cover through the co-op which will make available a range of choices of insurance policy. Individuals will make an annual choice between insurers. Their choice will be assisted by the co-op which will give advice and price a standard plan for its area. People who are self-sufficient would get back 50 per cent of the standard plan as a tax credit; people on benefit, 100 per cent. No one should face exclusions or limitations of coverage because of pre-existing conditions. The poorest people would be empowered to choose both doctor and hospital. Such a system would also avoid imposing costs on employers, an additional burden that could easily tip the balance in favour of re-location overseas.

Convert primary care trusts to mutuals

Another possibility would be to convert PCTs to mutual organisations owned by their members. At the minimum this would require direct representation of patients on the controlling body of the PCT, but it would be better to go a step further to create real ownership by giving members control of their share of the Treasury allocation to the PCT. Better still, members should be allowed to take this amount with them to another PCT to give trusts an incentive to provide a good standard of care.

Such a change would go some way towards empowering patients, but PCTs would still have cash-limited budgets set by central government. To overcome this problem, people need to be free to add to the funding available to their PCT, but how can such freedom be made compatible with social solidarity?

One method would be to let PCTs establish separate mutual funds for service development. Members could pay into the fund just as they pay into any savings account. Interest would be free of tax and payable so long as the capital were tied up for long enough to allow its use for investment in health facilities – perhaps until retirement age. Once the members reached the age of 65 the capital could be withdrawn or left to gather further interest. Each year huge amounts are invested in pensions and, if the tax regime for mutual health funds were the same as it is for pensions, it is possible that many people would be willing to invest in mutual health funds as a way of combining provision for retirement with support for the NHS. As the years passed and members grew older, money would start to be withdrawn from the mutual funds, but in the short run there will be a major growth in funding for the development of health care services. If we are to catch up with other European countries we need just such an immediate boost in funding.

An arrangement based on mutually-owned PCTs would be voluntary and potentially create a sense of genuine social solidarity – always promised by the NHS but never achieved.

Convert primary care trust to health maintenance organisations

The chief difficulty with proposals to mutualise PCTs (or hospitals) is that most doctors are unlikely to want to work for organisations run by consumers. For this reason it would be more realistic to convert PCTs into health maintenance organisations run by doctors. Patients should be free to switch to another PCT if dissatisfied and it may be possible to establish the mutual funds already discussed, so that additional funds can be raised quickly. But ownership and control of the PCT should lie with the doctors who work in it. In most markets for goods and services we do not rely on direct consumer representation on company boards to ensure good service, but rather on competition. Health care is no different.

Self-governing hospitals

It is now widely accepted that political involvement in hospital management has become counter-productive. Even the diehard apologists for the NHS at the King's Fund have come to this view in their recent report, despite clinging to reliance on taxation as the chief source of finance.

There is now a cross-party consensus in favour of establishing self-governing hospitals. Even Mr Milburn has announced that he is willing to take such ideas seriously. Ruth Lea, in this publication, advocates mutual ownership of hospitals and a loose coalition has been founded, co-ordinated by the New Economics Foundation, to increase awareness of public service organisations that are not in the public sector.

During Alan Milburn's speech to the New Health Network in January 2002, he said that 3-star trusts might become independent, non-profit organisations or Foundation Hospitals. This was all part of a search, he said, for a 'middle ground between state-run public and shareholder-led private structures'.

Several structures are already available: charities, companies limited by guarantee, mutuals, co-operatives and organisations founded by royal charter. Charities are run by trustees who can not benefit financially from the work of the charity. All assets must be used exclusively for charitable purposes and if the objects of the charity change then all donations must be used for a similar 'public' purpose. All changes require the permission of the Charity Commission. Unlike mutual organisations, there is no possibility of privatising the assets.

Mutuals are regulated by the Industrial and Provident Societies Acts and come in two main forms. Usually they are run for the benefit of members (such as a co-operative of farmers or workers). They can also be run for the benefit of the community. Friendly societies are similar but have separate legislation and may also be run for the members or for the benefit of other people.

There has been recent interest in creating a new structure, called a public interest company (PIC), an idea that draws partly on the American tradition of 'public benefit corporations'. The Public Management Foundation produced a report in June 2001 setting out the case for PICs. One of its authors, Paul Corrigan, subsequently became Mr Milburn's special adviser. The idea is to create a new kind of trading organisation whose character cannot be changed by simple resolution of shareholders, directors or members. Like a charity, it will be unable to alter its objects without permission from an independent regulator, but it will not have the tax breaks enjoyed by charities. Shareholders would hold only preference shares redeemable at face value. Trading surpluses would have to be ploughed back for the benefit of the public and not distributed to shareholders or anyone else. PICs would resemble mutual structures for the benefit of the community (currently registered under the Industrial and Provident Societies Acts) but would not be able to privatise the assets.

Another alternative that would not require legislation would be to give hospitals royal charters, like universities and many voluntary hospitals before nationalisation. Universities have the powers given them by the royal charter and nothing can be changed without the approval of the Privy Council. Like a charity, the assets cannot be privatised and must permanently be used for the public purpose stipulated in the royal charter. As a result, if you leave a hospital founded by royal charter some money in your will, you can be sure it will be used for health care and not find its way in someone else's pocket.

There is no need to invent new structures. The real challenge is to recognise that the creation of self-governing hospitals would achieve three vital ends. First, it would create competition and enhance the power of service users. Second, by ending public sector monopoly, it would permit the inventiveness and creativity that can only flourish in an open system. And third, it would help to rebuild the social fabric by providing outlets for goodwill and community service in every major town. Before nationalisation, the local hospital had long been able to unite people from all walks of life in a common cause. Everybody benefits if there is good health care near at hand and so any appeal for generosity of time or money draws on a unique blend of self-interest and altruism.

Conservatives used to be the champions of voluntary service and they used to understand its dual purpose as a means of providing better ways of meeting human needs and as a generator of independent organisations capable of serving as bastions against over-mighty government. It's time to re-awaken this dormant strand in Conservative thought and march towards the sound of gunfire.

Renewing Civil Society

Where will the money come from? One possibility would be to adapt tax systems found elsewhere in Europe. Germany, for example has a church tax which largely funds voluntary organisations.

Instead of paying a church tax, perhaps we should allow people to earmark part of their income tax for distribution to voluntary organisations. We might call it a civic responsibility tax. Income tax produces about £97 billion. If we allowed people to direct 10 per cent of their tax away from the Treasury to voluntary organisations, including schools and hospitals, the potential revenue would be nearly £10 billion.

There would have to be conditions. To receive civic responsibility taxes, organisations would need to be completely independent of the government. Receipt of government grants would disqualify them from receiving it. They would also need to be non-profit. In this manner taxpayers could divert their income tax from the Treasury to permit a truly independent sector to develop gradually. They would pay the same tax as before, but they could ensure that it is used for the common good.

Conclusion

The NHS is one of the biggest tests faced by the Conservatives. During Mr Hague's leadership it was argued that the NHS would always be a winning issue for Labour and that Conservatives would always lose out if they tried to tackle it. Labour, it was argued, would react by making false accusations that the cold-hearted Tories wanted to dismantle the NHS, leaving nothing in its place. And mud sticks.

True to form, Mr Blair has already started to use this kind of argument. But a false accusation is a false accusation and it is now widely accepted across the political spectrum that many other countries have found ways of combining social solidarity with consumer choice. There are several ways of doing it and reasonable people can disagree about the details, but if the Conservatives run away from the issue again, they will not deserve to be elected.

Social insurance systems

Lessons from Europe

Stephen Pollard

Nigel Lawson famously referred to the NHS as the English religion. For years, blasphemy was an offence punishable by ostracism from polite society. Conservatives spent the past twenty years thinking that the NHS could only ever be a vote loser, and that their best tactic was too keep shtum about it. Those of us who, whether Conservative or not, looked abroad and saw that, in what they delivered to patients, almost every other system was superior to the NHS, had either to keep quiet or be viewed as lunatics.

Today, at last, things have changed. It is now acceptable to question the very existence of a state-run, tax-funded, monopoly health care provider. And that means that, for the first time in two generations, it is possible to imagine a time when the UK has a health system of which it can be genuinely proud, because it is possible to imagine a time when we move towards a pluralistic healthcare system.

Almost everyone agrees, of course, that healthcare in the UK needs more money. The question isn't even now how much. The real questions are where should that money come from, and how should it be spent – a crucial change in the terms of the debate.

The Government's aim is to make the NHS more responsive to consumers. Hurrah for that. But is there anyone who seriously thinks that the most efficient, most convincing method for delivery is through a public sector monopoly, even if that public sector monopoly starts to commission some of its services from a variety of providers? The very notion would be absurd in any other area.

The second notion which needs to be dismissed is that there is any 'holy grail' of healthcare systems to which we can look for inspiration. There isn't. The fact that there are so many systems which provide a better service than the NHS does not mean that there is one which we can import, lock, stock and barrel. Firstly, healthcare systems are a product of history, culture and politics. Each country has its variety. And second, systems which score highly in one area often have huge flaws in another – such as France [*see below*]. But for all their different problems, that does not mean, of course, that we should not learn from then what we can do better, and how. The absence of a holy grail is not an argument against reform but in favour of it, not just in Britain but elsewhere, too.

I was once told by an American health care analyst that, in the US, consumers actually have huge power; they just think they have none. The exact opposite is true with the NHS: although British patients think they have enormous power, in practice they have none. That is why British patients who are treated abroad, as I was in France in July 2001, are struck at just how different the NHS is from the systems of our continental neighbours. One key reason for that is, of course, that in continental social insurance systems, the consumer is indeed boss, rather than merely the grateful recipient of whatever a generous government consents to allow us. (The generic phrase 'social insurance' can sometimes be misleading, since it implies one system, and one funding method. In fact each EU country has its own distinct system, some funded by wage deductions, some based on private insurance, some based on a mix. But it is nonetheless still useful to contrast 'social insurance' systems, where healthcare is delivered by competing independent organisations and funded by extra-tax contributions, with tax-funded state monopolies, such as the NHS.)

Whilst almost all healthcare systems have in common a large measure of taxpayer/public funding (even the US, often cited as a lunatic private model, has similar levels of tax funding to the EU: 45 per cent of US healthcare is tax funded), there are two obvious differences between the NHS and every other European system: they all have a much larger measure of private, non-tax, non-compulsory insurance spending than in UK; and they all have a variety of competing providers – some state, some private, some profit-making, some not-for-profit.

Last July's European Court of Justice decision, which effectively forced the government to allow British NHS patients to be treated abroad, is by far the most significant development in healthcare over the past few years. The numbers of patients involved will never be more than a few thousand. But their impact will be enormous. Soon, most of us will know of someone who has been treated abroad, and we will start to ask the obvious question: how come we can't treat our own patients, and they have spare capacity? There will be a wave of anger at the wanton waste of billions of pounds thrown at a dying NHS, to no discernible effect. And then it will be practical politics to point to other systems, and show how they succeed and why we don't.

Take France. Purely as a patient, devoid of any other responsibilities, France is near-perfect. The French system is relatively straightforward. Most of the French population are covered by social insurance. When they visit a doctor, they pay up front, and are then re-imbursed for (roughly – the exact amount depends on the technical specification of the doctor) three quarters of the total. 87 per cent of families also take out additional 'supplementary' insurance, which covers the remaining quarter of the bill. A typical supplementary plan will cost €75 a month for full family cover.

Those who are not covered by social insurance – the 820,000 'destitute', with an income of less than €6,500 a year – are covered by the Couverture Maladie Universelle. In addition, there is also a CMU supplementary scheme (used by 4,300,000) which takes care of the balance of any bills paid by social insurance.

When they are ill, French patients have a totally free choice in who they wish to see. If they want to visit a GP, they do so. If they want to see another GP, they can do so. If they would rather go straight to a specialist, they can. And again, as often as they wish. Waiting lists are almost unheard of, and hospitals are modern and amongst the best in the world.

But there is no such thing as a free lunch. Whilst it is true that the French get what they pay for (they spend 9.5 per cent of GDP on healthcare), it is also true that the French system is economically unsustainable.

In France, employers pay a 'social insurance' premium of 13 per cent of workers' salaries; employees pay an additional 7 per cent of their income. This is not, as the British Prime Minister repeatedly insists it is, tax. There is a critical difference. Instead of going to the Treasury, to be handed out at the Chancellor's pleasure, the money goes directly to an independent insurance agency, governed by a board with representatives from consumers, the trade unions and employer, which exists to represent consumers.

This has huge strengths, not the least of which is that it has led to a wide variety of providers, some public, some private, all of which compete for custom, and between which the social insurance agency makes no distinction. All that matters is that the patient gets the best.

But if Mr Blair is wrong to talk about the French system as if it relies on high tax funding – it is the non-tax revenue of social and supplementary insurance which gives it its strength, and which empowers the consumer – he is nonetheless right to point to a critical problem. The French model of social insurance, for all its strengths, represents a premium on jobs, which has a series of deleterious knock-on effects. A generation on, the French system will be facing its own crisis. GP remuneration, for example, is so poor that there is already a massive recruitment crisis, which is far worse than anything faced in the UK, where the problem is not recruitment but simply a cap on the numbers trained. The majority of French GPs receive €18.5 per consultation. And that is it. Thus the average GP salary is about €45,000 per annum, out of which has to be paid tax (at 54 per cent), pension, and all expenses and office costs.

The same is true in Germany, where 'social insurance' originated under Bismarck. Contributions are again compulsory. But unlike France, the highest earners can opt out of the system and choose to be covered entirely privately, an option which is taken up by 10 per cent – and rising. The overwhelming majority, however, join a sickness fund of their choice (unlike France, where there is only one, national, social insurance agency). A risk-adjustment formula transfers money from funds with healthier members to those with less healthy patients. The funds compete for members through price and the level of benefits offered. Contributions, which vary between funds, are split equally between employers and employees, and average 13.5 per cent of gross income. But, as in France, they have huge wage cost effects: the average German worker costs employers $26.90 an hour (of which 46 per cent goes towards welfare benefits); the average US worker, in contrast, costs $15.89 hour (of which 28 per cent goes towards welfare benefits).

So these social insurance systems are far from perfect

(although they are a lot less imperfect than the NHS). The same theoretical model (multiple payer systems, with costs paid by independent sickness funds paid for by a premium on wages) also operates, with wide differences in structure, in Austria, Belgium and the Netherlands. But theory and practice are rather different: for all the quality of the care, which is patients' prime concern, members usually have no idea about the size of their premium (which is set by the government) and more often than not pay nothing themselves beyond some kind of supplementary insurance. They thus have no incentive at all to keep costs down. And all such funds run enormous deficits, balanced by taxes.

But just as it is right to look at the downside, it is misleading, as opponents of change would have it, to pretend that they are inherent in social insurance. For one thing, premiums do not have to be paid by employers. They are not in Switzerland. The Swiss system is based on compulsory insurance, with competing insurers and minimal interference by the state. But because they pay their own premiums, consumers know precisely how much they are paying. Premiums are kept down by competition between the insurers.

One of the state's few roles is to provide targeted subsidies for those who cannot pay for their own insurance. If your premium exceeds between 8-10 per cent of your taxable income you are entitled to a subsidy. And in Ireland, as in Switzerland, insurers must offer a minimum level of benefits, with open enrolment, regardless of pre-existing conditions. Cover is lifelong so that, as people grow older and pose a greater cost threat to the system, they are not cut off.

The flexibility of the Swiss model, and the variety of insurance packages offered, means that the structure of the system is determined to a far greater degree than in other countries by the preferences of patients themselves. The Swiss model, of course, is like any other in that it is locally developed and large parts of it are relevant only to Switzerland. The high level of decentralization, for example, with 26 cantons in charge of hospital accreditation and finance, means that cantons learn from each other's successes and failures. It also has its flaws: those hospitals are state run, and often inefficient.

So we could not simply import the Swiss model. What works in one country would be totally unsuitable elsewhere. But there is no reason, other than politics, why we could not import our own version of its most relevant features. And one thing is clear: there is no successful healthcare system that does not involve a large measure of private contributions, and complementary, competing providers, some state, some private.

As my colleague, Paul Belien, has pointed out, whilst policy wonks too often analyse systems against perfect models, experience suggests that the complexity of health systems across the globe is unavoidable. Mostly, the complications derive from misguided attempts to correct the most pervasive law of public policy: the law of unintended consequences. New tranches of health reforms are often introduced to correct the shortcomings of the last set, creating illogical bundles of arrangements which depend on and contradict each other. Take France again, where the central principle of *lamedicine libérale* requires freedom of choice for patients, and where doctors are paid on a fee for service basis. To mitigate the effects of moral hazard caused by this payment method, there is a co-payment system. But this also undermines the other principle underpinning the French system – solidarity, so co-payments are insured so that their disproportionate effect is not too pronounced. But this undermines the ability to control moral hazard. And so on . . .

There is one further problem which needs to be considered when we are looking at alternative models of healthcare provision. Almost all EU healthcare is Pay As You Go – healthy young workers paying for the care of sick, usually older patients. They then rely on future generations to pay for theirs – 'solidarity', to use the preferred EU jargon. But demographic changes – a falling birth rate and growing life expectancy – will cause real problems. The EU Member States are demographically very similar. Birth rates are declining everywhere, and are much lower than reproduction rates, so that we can expect a negative growth in the total population, starting in 2010 in Germany, in 2014 in Spain and across the EU as a whole in 2020. The size of the over '60s sector, compared with the rest of the population, is projected to double across the EU, leading to significant rises in health expenditure in both the public and private sectors. Older people – especially those aged 80 years and above – incur expenditures per year and per capita on average eight or nine times higher than younger people. So just as we need more money to pay for care, so there will be fewer in absolute and relative numbers to pay for it. That means that either the level and quality of care will have to decline sharply, or premiums will have to rise astronomically. But the increase necessary for that to be sufficient is beyond the pale: in a tax-based system because of the impact on the overall tax burden; and in a wage-related system because of the changes in the contribution ratio and the side effects on unemployment.

The unspoken truth is that PAYG healthcare systems cannot last. Just as EU pensions are in crisis, so healthcare has to move towards some kind of funded arrangement. The NHS is not the only health system in crisis. Ours is merely more immediate.

Any party which is serious about reform, rather than tinkering at the edges, needs not only to address delivery and tax funding; it needs also to look at the whole question of Pay As You Go insurance, whether state or social, and the need for a funded system. Conservatives, of all people, should be aware of this, having managed a similarly revolutionary change in pension provision.

This will probably the most politically difficult of all changes. As I said at the beginning, the political climate has already been transformed, such that it is now possible to talk about replacing the NHS model without being pilloried. That is because, quite simply, patients are no longer prepared to be patient, and to put up with a service demonstrably and dangerously inferior to that offered elsewhere in Europe. The political consequence of that is that there is a desire for change. We are now in the middle of a practical experiment – whether the NHS's real problem is funding. If, after the massive spending boost it is receiving, the service is transformed, then reform will not be a practical proposition. But no one – not even, I suspect, Alan Milburn – really expects that to happen. At the end of this Comprehensive Spending Review period, the most likely outcome is that the extra billions of pounds spent will have bought no discernible improvement. And then it will be obvious to almost everyone that something has to change. In almost no other walk of life do we consider the state the most efficient spender of our money. Just as a monopoly state owned, tax funded grocer would cause chaos – just ask any Cuban for proof – so competition between Sainsbury and Tesco ensures that there is a sufficient supply of food, and that times of huge demand (such as Christmas) are not a problem, as they are for the NHS, but an opportunity. Patients are beginning to realise this, and to see that the person best placed to fund and choose his healthcare is the patient, not the Chancellor of the Exchequer and Secretary of State for Health.

That is the political opportunity for reformers.

Can the UK learn anything from the Stockholm health care transition programme?

Johan Hjertqvist

Introduction

In the welfare societies of tomorrow, services such as education and health-care must involve the consumer, ensuring that he or she can participate rather than be simply dictated to. And if the consumer is to be treated as a partner, he or she must have access to the best information available.

My analysis of the healthcare reforms that have taken place in Stockholm is made on this basis. The Stockholm Transition (as it is known here) has been neither perfect nor well-defined. Rather, it has been the basis of a more constructive discussion on the future of healthcare in Sweden.

The transformation in Stockholm has been going on for some ten years. How did it start? What have been the outcomes? And is there really something to brag about at international conferences?

I think so. The journey from a bureaucratic, production-based, centrally-funded, multi-tiered system to one that is, (hopefully) less regulated, consumer focused, efficiency rewarding and incentivised, has only just started. Nevertheless, the Stockholm transformation might – if I may use a somewhat strained (and dangerous) simile – be 'the new economy' of health care.

Is there a risk that it will flop? Yes, there is a risk, especially if the public lose faith or the politicians lose their will. It will be difficult to assess the outcomes. But I am in no doubt that, at the very least, there is no way back to the old kind of healthcare.

But change is certainly a very complicated and risky business, especially when dealing with such a huge structure, and especially when tools for measuring the result of change are still lacking.

A visit to Stockholm

The Stockholm Transition, which is receiving widespread attention, attracts an increasing number of international visitors. Having guided some of them and been interviewed by others, my impression is that they come for the following reason: you might be a politician from the UK, a journalist from the Netherlands, a manager from Canada, or a lobby group representative from Norway – regardless of background you are involved in a reform discussion at home. So you look around for inspiration.

The US? My God, everybody hates that system (or at least the general perception of it, including many Americans). The NHS

– 'the Mother of Public Health Care'? Ouch! No thanks, too many have already tried that one! Medical Savings Accounts in Singapore – well, a bit exotic, maybe. Are not those careful, reliable Scandinavians up to something? A bit of solidarity, a bit of public funding, a bit of public health?

Thank heavens, they are! In Stockholm – that must be worth looking at! Sweden – The number one Welfare State (well, at least up until 20 years ago). If they start transforming public health-care, it must be relevant. When is the next flight?

More seriously, what, in my view, is attractive and surprising to foreign observers is how a heavy, old-fashioned, and politically managed system can change. The idea is to open up the system to new incentives and operators while maintaining levels of funding, principles of equal access, public responsibilities and so on. You might even say (as I prefer to put it myself, nowadays supported by for example Tony Blair) that in order to safeguard public health care, you must 'modernise' the tools and conditions, otherwise you will fail, losing the support of your co-workers as well as public confidence. Reform or die!

What visitors to Stockholm can find is, for example:

- Incentives which address the need for productivity. Instead of central budgets, hospitals do not get compensation until they deliver. Competition for public contracts is open to great numbers of private, as well as public, providers.
- Market-oriented approaches. Hospitals are turned into limited companies, creating an opening for a more entrepreneurial approach

- A clear division between purchasers and providers, clarifying the responsibilities of each party (and ensuring the politicians leave the production side alone).
- Publicly employed personnel getting active legal and educational support to start their own companies, which can take over the operation of primary care clinics and other contracted facilities.
- A rapid expansion of Stockholm Council's consumer information, supporting active consumer behaviour and choice [www.vardguiden.nu], and which is said to be 'state of the art'.
- Far better access to healthcare than in other parts of Sweden, i.e. shorter waiting lists and a choice of providers.

To many visitors the Stockholm Transition is astonishing, based perhaps not on the hard evidence of outcomes but compared to the common view of Swedish healthcare as a system based on socialist values of 'solidarity,' 'equality,' and political control, values which have hitherto reduced essential modernisation to wishful thinking. The contrast with the actual situation in Stockholm is quite dramatic. It is an example of Swedish modernisation using tools of pragmatic co-operation between public and private initiatives.

Since the mid-90's (when Sweden entered the EU) things have been changing rapidly. The traditional power base of the Social Democrats, the TUC and other 'traditionalist' strongholds opposes change, so the official view is that everything must stay the same. Equality and solidarity must rule, public welfare will remain. But below the surface modernisation is underway, questioning most parts of the traditional 'Swedish model.'

User fees for health and dental care are rising. Competition among providers for public contracts is very tough. A large number of local authorities, including cities with a leftist majority, use competitive tendering of contracts as a means of lowering costs in welfare facilities such as nursing homes and psychiatric care. The same goes for councils, which, step by step, are opening primary care for contracted entrepreneurs (a process explicitly welcomed by the Minister of Health). In the labour market, the TUC heartland and consequently less reformed, Manpower and other for-hire agencies are growing. In healthcare few under-staffed hospitals can turn down offers to hire doctors and nurses.

Stockholm leads this movement. I am convinced that other councils and cities eventually will follow. There are no alternatives to modernisation.

A different kind of argument

But if you listen to the Swedish political debate, or rather quarrel, the arguments sound quite different. There is little room for this kind of long-term analysis or for intellectual reflection. British readers are probably only too familiar with the phenomenon. But what might add some flavour to the Swedish election debate (which ends in September 2002) is the fight on healthcare policy between the national Social Democratic government and its regional Centre-Right opponent in the Stockholm Greater Council.

Born out of frustration

The road to the Stockholm Transition started in the late 1980s, when frustrated council politicians felt a need to reform the management of the healthcare system. Or, more correctly, they saw it as a matter of life or death to regain control over hospitals that were delivering less and less but costing more and more.

You could have described the healthcare situation in Stockholm like this (which goes for Sweden in general, as well): After three decades of rapid economic growth the Swedish economy was slowing down. But the publicly funded systems were used to ever increasing funding. For every extra injection of tax money, waiting-lists grew more and more.

Since the central budget system rewarded the least efficient clinics, where the worst queues were to be found, much more creativity was directed to funding manipulation than to increased productivity. Sound familiar?

By the end of the 1980′s the time was ripe to take more radical action. An informal coalition of Moderates and Social Democrats in Stockholm started to introduce health care reforms. Literally overnight a Diagnosis Related Group system was introduced, taking its inspiration from the US. DRGs are systems used to measure what resources are necessary for a wide range of treatments. In the Stockholm purchaser-provider system the DRG sets the price for many of the contracted services.

Out went central budgets and in came a compensation system, where the hospitals were paid according to what they really delivered, not according to what the budget said that should produce. Close to 500 'products' were defined by the DRG price-list, and prices were gradually reduced to reflect the appropriate level of compensation.

The outcome of this reform was at least twofold. The mentality of hospital managers changed dramatically. And as a result productivity figures rose dramatically.

Sound incentives pay

Being a strong believer in the power of incentives I am happy to say that the hospital staff were extremely quick in adapting to the new conditions.

The aim of the leadership of Stockholm Council was to boost the efficiency of critical services and so get rid of tiresome waiting lists. Suddenly the old formula was of no value to old-fashioned managers: pointing at a long waiting list as an argument for another budget increase was no longer a good idea. Instead the name of the game was to attract purchasers willing to pay for a higher number of treatments, and so increase patients' access.

Central budgets give the staff a tool to reduce costs when the economy gets tough. That means cutting down on activity, closing down units, postponing treatments. If you are, instead, paid a fixed price for every item you deliver it is natural to attack budget deficits by increasing income, i.e. raising production. You think about how to increase quality, lower prices, improve access, in other words how to become more competitive – a 180 degree about-turn compared to yesterday's mentality.

What about productivity, then? In the first year of the Stockholm reform (1991) it increased by 19 per cent. The clearcut incentive corresponded very well with the political signals – that the one who delivered instead of spending time in meetings and on paper work would get a premium. Waiting times were generally very much reduced. The success was almost too great, in the sense that the increase in care and operations provoked increased spending.

The DRG-system provided a new way to plan and pay for additional care. But that was not enough to create a market environment, to break up the traditional bureaucratic way of acting. From 1996 onwards, purchasers and providers were separated. This split was undertaken so that the politicians could focus on representing the citizens simply by formulating visions for health care policy. In withdrawing from the production side, the politicians wanted to signal that finding the practical solutions as well as handling the given budget was a professional manager's matter.

The Council's new strategy was to treat every producer equally, opening up the system to large-scale competition. The privately owned providers already knew how to operate in this system. But the council-run competitors did not.

To behave like a player in the marketplace you need the appropriate mental mindset. By transforming the six publicly owned emergency hospitals into limited companies, though still controlled by the council, the Centre-Right regional government wanted to combine decentralisation with business-like thinking. Professional company boards and managements could act highly independently within a distinctive framework.

This approach was formulated in 1998, when the Moderate-led coalition had returned to power in the metropolitan area. After a four-year period of Social Democratic rule which neither advanced nor revoked the reforms, the Moderates were ready for a big step forward: private contractors were invited to take over the operation of every publicly owned health-care facility outside the hospitals. That was a radical leap.

Remarkable success

The Moderates could by then look back on the successful reorganization of the Stockholm healthcare policy. As early as in 1994 one emergency hospital – the St Goran – became a limited company (owned by the Council) as part of a restructuring process. The outcome was an impressive rise in productivity by roughly 40 percent. This achievement invited further progress.

Competition in the contracting process, which had started in the early 1990's, had resulted in significantly reduced costs for several services, such as laboratory work, X-ray treatment, and the ambulance service. In fact many of these first tender agreements resulted in cost reductions of between 10 and 40 per cent. Some of the reductions proved sustainable, while others showed rather that large companies knew how to manipulate prices. New producers entered the market, adding pluralism to the group of providers.

According to researchers at the Stockholm School of Economics, county councils implementing a purchaser-provider-split have increased the efficiency of their health care systems by in average 13 percent compared with 'unreformed' councils.

Another outcome was a rapidly increasing number of primary care suppliers operated by private contractors. Today 40 percent of primary care is operated by private contractors. If one looks at the total health-care system in the metropolitan area the share is 23 percent – compared to an average of just 7 per cent in the whole country.

Among the private providers the majority have only been recently established – most of the companies were founded during the 1990's. In Stockholm there is a large proportion of former public sector employees, who were actively encouraged by the Council to take over primary health clinics and mother and child-care units. To become an entrepreneur is an attractive opportunity for public employees today.

The trade unions and consumers are happy

To the astonishment of foreign observers the healthcare trade unions have supported these reforms. This is rational behaviour; because for the first time health-care workers have access to alternatives to public employment.

By using this new freedom to 'vote with their feet' all categories of personnel have improved their working conditions substantially faster than in other parts of Sweden. Between 1996 and 1998 nurses received a salary increase of 17 percent – more than twice what they had got before. (Lifting the general compensation level is a necessary step in recruiting and keeping health-care personnel.)

A number of surveys show that private producers have a good record in terms of employee satisfaction. The private managers are more competent and available. The employees understand and share the goals of the enterprise (far from always the situation in publicly operated units).

In addition, frequent polls say consumers rank privately-run parts of the health-care supply higher than their public alternatives. They are said to adapt better to consumer conditions in finding new ways to tackle problems. When staff take over publicly managed units the consumers generally give the new operators better scores than before.

Things are getting tougher

Since 1998 things have become more complicated, partly due to diverse opinions inside the majority coalition, partly because the transformation of such a large, complex structure might have needed a more consistent strategy.

On the plus side, there has been the sale of the St Goran hospital to Capio, a listed healthcare company well known in the UK. This example is a good benchmark, delivering high quality services at 15 per cent lower costs than the average in other Stockholm emergency hospitals. This hospital operates within the public system under the same rules as those owned by the Council. The St Goran has the same mix of patients and as yet no evaluation has found signs of 'cream-skimming.' The management is not allowed to turn away complicated cases.

However, because of lack of support from the coalition partners, the Moderates could only support the effort to turn the remaining hospitals into companies owned by the Council. Internal resistance has, alas, severely delayed even this development, causing confusion about the strategy and the sustainability of the reform effort.

Supreme access

The most outstanding achievement of all these reforms has been patient access.

The waiting time for an examination or treatment is much shorter than in other parts of Sweden. The most striking contrast is to be found in a comparison to the least reformed county councils, i.e. where leftist 'traditionalists' are most powerful. Every council today 'guarantees' treatment within three months. But it is only in Stockholm that a patient can rely on this commitment.

Outside the metropolitan area you must often wait for a year to get a hearing device (four weeks in Stockholm), up to two years for a knee plastic (two–ten weeks) and ten months for hernia surgery (two–four weeks). We are not, of course, talking about emergency cases, but other patients are supposed to be able to wait – some voluntarily, but many others paying the price of long duration in sick leave, pain, and a reduced quality of life.

It is worth stressing that Stockholm offers a better access for the same – or sometimes lower – price per capita as under-achieving councils.

A new perspective

The consumer will look upon healthcare as one of many sets of services. Their judgement will be based on how quickly and competently demands can be dealt with. In order to succeed health-care organisations must implement incentives which drive and develop new sophisticated services. They will certainly not succeed just by abandoning bureaucratic principles in favour of consumer-market influence.

We can identify such a process in the Stockholm region. The core change is the introduction of rational incentives to improve performance, not only in economic terms but also in services to the consumer, in market information, and in conditions for employees. This means that the monopoly must be abandoned in favour of pluralism, starting with the production side.

In the long run the purchaser-monopoly will be challenged throughout Sweden. Taxes will not be enough to meet the costs and consumers who can pay extra money will demand influence. There will eventually be private insurance or a breakthrough for savings accounts.

Something to learn?

From a policy point of view, what are the lessons from Stockholm?

Do not underestimate the complexity of reform. In

Stockholm I suspect that the Council coalition from the start did not carry out the necessary strategy implementation. The process was driven rather by intuition than by knowledge. Pressing the start button is only the first step – after that you have to correct and re-adjust the next steps for many years.

Go for radical action. In this respect politics is not a perfect environment. Compromise might be tempting but it is dangerous. If you calculate that success requires a certain input of investment or compensation, it is a risky business to reduce that effort to please coalition partners or opponents. In that case you would face a lose-lose situation. The radical empowerment of the consumer by giving her, not the bureaucrats, the purchasing power was never part of the Centre-Right agenda. It has stopped at simply handing over control of much of the healthcare system to private producers. To me, that has been a strategic mistake.

Centrally funded healthcare systems will be driven by perverse incentives (such as encouraging long waiting lists). On the other hand, when you start paying for the services that are delivered, you encourage appropriate incentives. Building a sound, logical incentive structure is one of the most important things. That means, first and foremost, to make the purchaser see the advantages of buying, not details, but a good overall outcome for the consumer. The provider must be able to rely on the fact that efficiency will always be better paid than inefficiency (which astonishingly often is not the case). And both parties must understand that, in business, agreements are valid (in politics the culture is different).

Here the political management must *never* compromise or hesitate – if they do, nobody will believe in real change! Then you will go on doing things the old way.

You cannot 'play market.' If you really want to take advantage of the power of competition – let providers compete. If not, don't give them a false impression. If you instead prefer a co-operative outcome, make that clear from the beginning. Accept the result, even if it rocks the boat. Otherwise there will be no offers next time.

Focus your attention on how to achieve the desired outcome. In Stockholm everyone has been saying that for years. But as long as you lack the system to evaluate results which separate the bad from the good, you will just go on talking. As I have said before, the consumer must play a vital part. How can you think of measuring the outcome without involving the consumer? Here radical steps must be taken.

I should like to add another piece of experience-based advice: *trust people*. People react to incentives. If they notice that increased productivity pays, they will perform. If, instead, you signal that bad access will provide more funding, the result will be very long waiting lists.

My final message is a brutal one: Do not expect any reform to permanently reduce net healthcare costs. The combination of increased individual demand, negative demography, and scientific advance will increase costs. You can affect the speed and the cost level in individual segments, but not the overall costs. Keep that in mind before setting your goals for reform. (We may, on the contrary, start thinking of health care costs rather as an investment, which reflects people's priorities for a good quality of life.)

A general cost reduction is one thing; getting more and better services for every penny is something else. The latter must be a central aim for change, attacking the costs of inefficiency and bad quality. If the Stockholm Council can fit the pieces together, the chances for a successful reform of health-care procedures will be good.

A tough but necessary journey

It will, alas, take some time to prove that you are right, when you start to turn the organisation upside down by paying for quality instead of quantity, and by starting to account for and evaluate strange new things, such as consumer satisfaction, before the amount of X-ray films used. You must ask yourself if you are tough enough to drive the process of change until success can be proven.

I do hope that you are not getting the impression that my advice to you is to avoid reform. On the contrary!

How can you avoid taking action, when you know that tens of thousands of patients ought to get faster treatment, that tens of thousands of old people suffer from the lack of co-operation between the different bodies of the health care apparatus, that just as many people of active age could get back to an active life if rehabilitated, and that new ways of working in health-care are urgent in order to improve the energy and motivation of the staff? All this and much more could be done if we can make the health-care system work more efficiently. This is a very good reason for change.

But, as a visit to Stockholm will show, this is not an easy journey.

The future of general practice

Dr Jonathan Reggler

Introduction

The National Health Service is virtually the last organisation in this country that is run in a way that Stalin would both have understood and approved. Run by central command and control, the NHS is to health care what British Leyland was to the motor industry and a nationalised BT was to the telephone industry. If the introduction of mobile phones had been organised by the NHS there would be only one tariff, twice as expensive as anything on the continent yet always displaying 'system busy' whenever you try to make a call.

The NHS is overly bureaucratic and appallingly politicised. None of the political parties can be exempted from blame. In power, the Conservatives lacked the political courage to apply their belief in individual responsibility to health care. A party that successfully showed the nation the value of free enterprise left the principles upon which the NHS was built virtually untouched. The NHS internal market was no more than a sop to its own supporters, a *faux* market still hamstrung by the real customer's inability to take part in transactions.

The difference between equity and egalitarianism

It is fair that those who are not able to afford the necessities in life – food, shelter, clothing, healthcare – should be assisted by those who can. This is what the welfare state is for. An important source of difficulties in any discussion about the NHS is that socialists – who are in the main egalitarians – have succeeded in persuading most Britons that they are interested in fairness. In fact the socialist creed of egalitarianism demands that everyone is treated the same, which is very different.

Confusing the principles of equity and equality has led to the lower standards of the NHS when compared with other first world nations' health services. We have a 'one size fits all' service. Any move to improve services in one area risks the charge of developing an 'unacceptable' two-tier service. Improvements have to wait until they can be engineered across the whole system. This is usually either impossible or at best very slow.

Why general practice matters

It may not be immediately apparent why GPs are such an important part of the system of medical care in the UK.

A GP is responsible for co-ordinating a patient's care and acting as their advocate and guide through the medical system. All other doctors who see the patient are required by the General Medical Council to write to the GP with details of the results of examinations and the treatment provided. The GP therefore holds the patient's lifelong clinical record, passing it to the next GP when the patient moves or chooses to change doctor. This aids continuity of care.

Another important function of the GP is to act as the main gatekeeper to secondary care. The gatekeeper role may appear to be about stopping patients from seeing specialists when they want to. In fact, the gatekeeper role protects patients. Specialists mainly see patients who have already been 'sieved' by GPs trained specifically to recognise serious illnesses in the much larger number of mild conditions presented to them by patients. If specialists saw patients without referral they would be overwhelmed by the numbers trying to see them. Waiting lists would become even longer. More importantly, many patients would find themselves being overinvestigated and overtreated for conditions which a GP would have recognised as less serious.

The problem with general practice

General practice has become an unpopular specialty for young doctors. The NHS general practitioner service is under enormous pressure. Thanks to chronic underfunding of the infrastructure of general practice and long-term planning errors there is now a crisis in the service. General practitioners' morale is low. Last summer 86 per cent of the 66 per cent of GPs who voted in a BMA ballot said that they would consider resigning from the NHS if their contract was not improved.

Recruitment is very poor. The government declared in the NHS Plan that 2000 more GPs would be recruited by 2004. The

BMA's General Practitioners Committee and the Royal College of General Practitioners calculated that if the NHS Plan's promises were kept, slightly more than 10,000 extra full-time GPs would be needed.[1] A mere 310 additional GPs have been recruited since the NHS Plan was published in July 2000 and this is simply a head count. Many of the newcomers are part-time.

Retention of GPs is also a problem. Senior GPs are retiring early and younger GPs are already planning their escape. A national survey of Britain's GPs last year revealed that whilst only 17 per cent of GPs originally intended retiring before 60 years of age, 48 per cent now plan to do so.[2]

A demographic time bomb is also about to go off. In the 1960s and 1970s large numbers of doctors from the Indian subcontinent were encouraged to come to the UK to set up GP practices. Many will retire over the next five years.[3] Their practices are predominantly in deprived areas and replacing them will be extremely difficult. There are already places such as the North East of England where deprived areas are seriously under-doctored because of the difficulty of recruiting GPs. Rural areas face the same problem. Even in the leafy shires vacant posts which would previously have attracted dozens of applicants now receive barely a handful and sometimes none at all. Practices in the home counties are closing their lists because they have failed to recruit GPs.

Why is general practice an unpopular career?

Work intensity

GPs are working more intensely than ever. Welcome medical advances mean that whereas previously there was little that a doctor could offer a patient who had had a heart attack or who had developed diabetes, for example, there are now proven interventions that are likely to lengthen a patient's life. Few are one-off episodes of care, however. A common feature of effective medical treatment is the need to review patients more frequently than before. Twenty years ago, 5–7 minutes with the GP was all a patient needed. At the beginning of the 21st century a ten minute appointment is woefully inadequate to deal with many individual problems, let alone the two or three that many patients now ask their GP about.

Failure to fund general practice infrastructure

The infrastructure of general practice has been ignored or even wilfully attacked with the diversion of funds intended for staff in particular siphoned off to bale out other parts of the NHS. The progressive underfunding of infrastructure means that many practices are now reducing staff numbers when they should be increasing them.

State control

Organisations controlled by the State are clumsy. They usually have no effective fine control and little flexibility. The more rigid the control, the more likely it is that attempts to improve things will lead to unforeseen problems elsewhere because the system is unable to manage out new problems in a flexible manner.

The NHS is highly politicised, and ministers constantly interfering with it because of politically damaging stories in the press and a belief that active hands-on micromanagement of the service is needed to control the situation.

Numerous targets are introduced and hurdles put in front of GPs in the misguided belief that jumping them will improve standards of practice. Perverse incentives often develop. Targets for childhood immunisations, which were introduced by the Conservatives, lead to GPs sometimes removing 'refusers' from their lists if a target is likely to be missed. GPs have become adept at responding creatively to demands for information that proves that they are meeting other government targets. They have no qualms about this as the targets are often nonsensical. Managers at local primary care groups and trusts do not question the response and not infrequently encourage obfuscation as all they want is to be able to report to the next layer of management that their own targets have been achieved.

Thus a 'virtual NHS'[4] is created which has little relation to the real one. It is the virtual NHS which ministers are told about by senior managers and Department of Health officials. Although ministers know this NHS is a house built of straw it suits their purpose to trumpet its reported 'successes'.

Capitation-based payments

Rising workload is frequently cited by GPs as a major reason for discontent. Combined with the introduction of medical advances, the mainly capitation-based NHS system of paying GPs means workload rises without a proportionate increase in pay. If the problem of rising but unremunerated workload is not overcome in the future no amount of other fixes will reverse the decline in general practice's popularity as a career.

Innovation suppressed

Many GPs want to develop additional skills such as minor surgery, ultrasound scanning, acupuncture, osteopathy, psychotherapy and so on. It is in the nature of all professionals to seek to expand their skills and capabilities. However there is no financial incentive for GPs to do so as the NHS will not usually pay them for providing additional services. A few GPs will carry on regardless. Most will simply stay on the narrow tracks of NHS general practice.

This happens less in European countries where State control of general practice is less complete and where mixed funding exists. Patients receive public subsidies for some of their medical costs but are also able to contribute extra funds where they wish. European family doctors are quick to use new technologies and to develop new skills, often dealing with patients who in the UK have to be referred to hospital. Simple market economics encourages them to do so.

Change fatigue

Change in the NHS is not new but the NHS has been in a state of almost permanent flux since the Labour government took office. As soon as GPs have grasped the basics of the new 'rules', they change. It is demoralising to work in a system where new ways of working are constantly being invented, particularly when an objective assessment of the changes leads most GPs to the view that they are politically motivated, provide little or no improvement, and often worsen the situation.

Funding general practice (and the rest of the NHS)

The reliance on a free at the point of access system is a real problem for the NHS although it is popular with patients and also with doctors who, most having only ever practised in the NHS, are uncomfortable charging patients for medical services. However, GPs are increasingly finding that too many patients do not value that which is free, their approach to the NHS being that it is there to serve even their smallest need or desire. This would be fair enough in a system in which they had to pay for services but in a cash-limited free-at-the-point-of-access service it is disastrous. Personal responsibility is unpopular and patients attend GPs' surgeries ever more often with minor symptoms which previously they would rightly have ignored or at least given the chance to improve.

The effect of paying fees

In many countries co-payments (also called access fees, user fees or patient charges) are used as a safe and effective way of reducing access in systems that need to limit the demands made of them. The classic study of the effect of co-payments on patient behaviour, the Rand study, showed that they reduce demand without adverse effects on health

This randomized experiment addressed two key questions in health care financing: how much more medical care will people use if it is provided free of charge, and what are the consequences for their health? The researcher found that in plans that reimbursed a higher proportion of the bill, patients used substantially more services – indeed, those who paid nothing used 40 percent more services than those required to pay a high deductible – but the effect on the health of the average person was negligible.[5]

Paying a fee or co-payment empowers patients as those paying to access a service are much more likely to want to influence the way it is provided. Furthermore they will do so not as a supplicant in a 'free' system, relying on their 'rights', but as a consumer/customer. This produces much healthier relationships between doctors and their patients.

Taxation

Most politicians, including many Conservatives, assert that general taxation is the best way to raise funds for the NHS.

Relying on taxation to fund the NHS whilst preventing patients from contributing additional funds may be progressive and appeal to the British sense of fair play, but it does not work.

Funding is never sufficient. The reason is simple. People accosted by pollsters in the street adopt the role of 'concerned citizens' when asked about funding the NHS. They respond accordingly and call for more taxation. However, when in 'electorate' mode, the adult population regards increased taxation as anathema. Interestingly, recent surveys of public opinion show that dissatisfaction with the NHS has reached such a level that even concerned citizens are no longer willing to throw more money at it in the form of taxation, recognising that it is the system and not simply funding levels which are at fault.

What I would do if I were health secretary – rescuing British general practice

What is needed?

Any change to the system of general practice in the UK must do the following:

For patients

1 Give patients more time with their GP.
2 Give patients more choice. Patients need real choice in terms of the services GPs offer. To achieve this, GPs must be able to respond according to the usual commercial rules governing demand, supply and price.
3 Help patients see their GP at times which are more convenient for them. The current system of paying GPs makes the provision of additional non-office hours of opening very unattractive. Patients should expect to be offered a wider range of opening times but GPs should expect to be able to benefit

financially from doing so. Under a state system which shuns the market approach to the provision of services it is apparently improper to do this.

For GPs

1 Encourage quality. Put at its simplest this means giving GPs more time with each patient.

2 Either safely reduce demand for services by patients or make concerns about demand less relevant by encouraging improved recruitment and retention.

3 Make income workload sensitive.

4 Enable GPs to increase income.

5 Let GPs regain control of their professional lives. Not to do so will make it impossible to improve morale. A weak profession is attractive only to a short-sighted government.

For health services

1 Increase the proportion of gross domestic product spent on health care.

2 End excessive political interference.

How to do it

The key to rescuing British general practice (and the rest of health care) is to remove it from excessive political control and to allow it to operate in a system which is market-orientated at the sharp end even if patients are later assisted by reimbursement of some or all of their costs. Patients need to be allowed to operate as consumers.

New cardinal rules

There should be three rules for state involvement in healthcare:

1 The State should only partially fund health care, probably through part reimbursement of direct costs or of insurance premiums,

2 The State should not commission services except perhaps in deprived areas,

3 The State should not provide services through any organisation, local or national.

Future funding models

The following two models of funding healthcare are applicable to all health care services although their effects on general practice are examined here. When combined with adequate safeguards for those with the lowest incomes, both would produce the required effect of increasing funding in general practice whilst also improving standards and improving patient choice. Both would increase the independence of general practice, encouraging innovation and the development of improvements within the specialty in a manner that is not possible in a State-controlled monopoly service.

Model 1: non-compulsory risk-based personal health insurance

Patients would be free to choose either to insure themselves against the cost of general practitioner care or to pay out-of-pocket expenses as they arise.

GPs would set their own fees in competition with other GPs. The government would set, through negotiations with representative GP organisations such as the BMA and the

Independent GPs Association, the level of fees which it would pay GPs for services rendered to patients deemed unable to afford personal medical insurance.

GPs would be free to choose whether to see patients under these terms. Exempt patients would be free to choose to see GPs who charged more than the government fee, paying the difference through out-of-pocket payments. There would be political pressure on the government not to set the fee levels too low, as this would lead to general practitioners choosing not to practise in more deprived areas.

Model 2: compulsory community-rated health insurance

Health insurers would be required by law to provide policies that deliver a standard level of health care to all policyholders. Patients would be able to add extra levels of cover for higher premiums. The lowest level of medical cover available would equate to that currently available through the NHS.

Premiums would be community rated, with all members of the community paying the same premium for the standard level service, to prevent those with chronic health problems being disadvantaged. Companies would not be permitted to exclude individuals on the grounds of medical history.

All citizens would be required to take out health insurance although they could opt out of the compulsory community rated health insurance system and purchase standard risk-based health insurance.

The government would pay the premiums of those judged

unable to pay themselves. This should include people on low-income benefits but exemption should not automatically include all groups currently exempt from prescription charges.

General practitioners and GP practices would negotiate with insurance companies either individually or through organisations such as the BMA and the Independent GPs Association to agree the level of fees for items of service. Whilst GPs may choose to accept the agreed fee as full and complete payment for services, they would be free to charge fees greater than this amount, the patient paying for the difference as an out-of-pocket expense. This would allow flexibility locally, with GP practices able to increase income to cover, for example, higher staff salaries in areas such as the South East.

Funding the system

The government would have two options.

Option 1

It could maintain the current level of spending on the public provision of health care and divert the funds currently spent on general practice into reimbursement of patients' secondary care costs (whether insurance-based or otherwise) and the provision of general practitioner services to those citizens who will be exempt from fees or premiums. All other citizens would be asked to fund their general practice insurance out of their income. On the island of Guernsey, where the NHS does not exist and most residents take out personal medical insurance cover, general practice cover costs about £48 per month for a family of four in 2001.[6] This would ensure a significant increase in the total level of spending in the UK on healthcare, allowing UK citizens to obtain the levels of service that are customary in countries such as France and Germany.

Option 2

The government could opt to pay a proportion of non-exempt citizens' general practice insurance premiums under either of the systems outlined above. Insurers would apply for reimbursement of a set amount based on validated policyholder rolls. This would encourage citizens to take out insurance even under the non-compulsory system, as their costs would be subsidised.

The effects of change – consequences for patients and general practitioners

Better choice

Both funding models outlined above would benefit patients. GPs would attract patients to their practices by offering services that patients want rather than services which anonymous NHS planners decide patients should have. Competition between practices would bring patients easier access, more comfortable surroundings, more time with their doctor, and higher clinical and outcome standards. At the same time good GP practices would be rewarded with increased income. This would allow practices to employ extra GP assistants and locums as well as improving the pay of GPs and their staff.

Valuing the service and coping with demand

A major positive feature of out-of-pocket and insurance-based systems is that patients value the service more than is the case in the UK, and they access healthcare more carefully.

In the NHS the problem of 'demand management' exercises doctors and managers. The concept is one that only really exists in free or excessively subsidised services. It is therefore important in the NHS. For patients, demand management really only means having one's wish to quickly see a doctor thwarted. For NHS GPs and their practice managers their inability to manage demand is a real problem. Demand for services increases steadily yet the numbers of doctors is increasing only very slowly.

If a 'fee for service' approach to medical care existed in the UK, whether paid for through out-of-pocket payments, voluntary insurance or compulsory community-rated social insurance, then there would be an expansion of general practice alongside a fall in the numbers of consultations being demanded of GPs (as shown by the Rand study). The expansion would come through more time being spent with each patient during each consultation. The improved working conditions, although combined with probably only a small increase in income (mirroring the dentists, who have seen average incomes rise hardly at all but working conditions improve considerably when they have moved out of the NHS and into private practices) would lead in turn to better recruitment and retention. Younger GPs who have removed themselves prematurely from the workforce would return. In time 'demand management' would become a term of historical interest only.

Reduced State interference

The government would lose its role in commissioning and providing services. History shows that governments are not good at either task; neither are organisations under their direct control, such as the NHS.

Keeping what works

When change happens it is important not to lose what works in the old system.

The referral system, which allows specialist services not to be overwhelmed and which protects patients from excessive investigation and treatment should be encouraged to remain.

Continuity of care and the maintaining of a lifelong medical record by GPs should also be encouraged.

Both these aims can be achieved through simple pricing mechanisms. This is easiest in a system of compulsory community-rated social insurance in which reimbursement occurs but insurance companies would almost certainly find the idea useful when determining the levels of co-payments under a system of voluntary insurance.

The continuation of the need for a patient to be referred by a

GP to a consultant should be achieved by having a higher level of reimbursement of fees incurred when seeing a specialist if the patient's own GP referred him. Continuity of care by GPs would be encouraged by having a higher level of fee reimbursement if a patient is seen at the GP practice at which he is registered.

---

1 Joint position statement on the general practitioner workforce, BMA/Royal College of General Practitioners, 19 December 2000.

2 National Survey of GP Opinion, General Practitioners Committee, BMA 2001.

3 Retrospective analysis of census data on general practitioners who qualified in South Asia: who will replace them as they retire? Donald H Taylor Jr and Aneez Esmail, BMJ 1999;318:306–10.

4 The term 'virtual NHS' was first used in this context by Professor Brian Salter in his paper *Trust me, I'm a doctor* , University of East Anglia, October 2000

5 'Free for All? Lessons from the RAND Health Insurance Experiment'. Newhouse, Joseph P., and the Insurance Experiment Group, Cambridge, Mass.: Harvard University Press, 1993.

6 The Guernsey Option Jonathan Reggler, Independent General Practitioners Association, 2001.

In my dreams

From life at the front line

Dr Kate Pickering

The front line of our NHS is the individual patient. Strange statement, I hear you say – surely it's the GP surgery or the hospital A&E, not the patients themselves? However, for those of us who are at the front line of the NHS – and I mean all the doctors, nurses, phlebotomists, physios, occupational therapists, paramedics, cleaners: the list goes on – the patient is the reason for us all to exist; therefore it is the time that we spend with the patients which matters the most.

For those of us who have been on the receiving end of the NHS, it is the time that the clinicians spend with us which matters to us the most. This is because that is our treatment, and when we are ill we are all vulnerable, and we all need time and attention. This valuable time with the patients and their treatments must be the priority.

Unfortunately, at present this isn't the case. Whether it's the dirty hospitals, lack of secretarial support or postcode lotteries, the NHS today and life at the front line goes on, despite the chaotic and crumbling structure which surrounds it. The system is quite simply creaking and relying on the goodwill of those at the front line to do a bit more, and then another bit more, and then a bit extra still. Goodwill was abundant in the NHS of the past, but in today's NHS where there are more administrators than hospital beds, where there is strangling red tape to be contended with, where the hospitals are dirty, where the canteens are closed during the night, and where the consultants have to share secretaries and offices, the goodwill from these teams has been exhausted. The clinicians are thoroughly fed up, morale is at an all time low, and management is thrashing around, politically driven, to achieve the government's election pledges. All this does is focus priority away from patient care. Poor clinicians, poor patients.

At present, all of our NHS failings are being blamed on lack of funding. Those of us at the front line are really fed up with this excuse. The real problem is the totally chaotic NHS management structure, which has changed constantly over the last 10 years. I believe that it is time for the government to de-politicise our NHS and take a few steps back. The NHS is heading towards the cliffs, and the only way that we can change this is by putting those at the front line in charge. It is only by putting the patients and the clinicians at the heart of the NHS that we can get the NHS back on a path of excellence. Excellent facilities for the clinicians, excellent facilities for teaching and research, excellent care for the patient.

I see the NHS as having three main roles. The first – and to the outside world most important – of these roles is to treat and prevent illness within the UK. The other two, which are often forgotten but which are equally as important, are training and research. We are currently facing a shortage of both doctors and nurses, and it is vital that we continue our world-envied training and teaching. To complement this, it is vital to encourage medical research at its highest levels. This is how we will keep world-class leaders in medical research and teaching in Britain and build on our reputation as a country at the forefront of medicine.

How do we do this? Well, I believe that we were on the right track in the 1990s. Margaret Thatcher had won the economic argument of the seventies and eighties, and by 1990 the economy was strong. The Conservatives at that time introduced the ideas of fundholding and trust hospitals: the first attempt for a long time to get the clinicians to be accountable for budgets, and therefore the care of their patients. The element of competition was thereby introduced, the idea being that competition would drive up standards. I believe the Conservatives made a particularly bad job of explaining these reforms to the public, which meant that the public as a whole rejected them. Competition was seen as being divisive, instead of liberating and empowering. This was not improved by parts of the medical and nursing establishment, who threw their hands up in horror stating that they were not managers.

For those doctors and nurses who did get involved in the reforms, the experience was, in retrospect, a rewarding one for themselves clinically as they were able to do their jobs better. It was also rewarding for the patients as the professionals were able to tailor the care provided to their patients' specific needs. However, these reforms were unfortunately hampered by some mistakes: the large privatisation contracts for cleaning and the closure of hospital beds before the community care side was sorted out were just two.

These mistakes never got a chance to be corrected: by then New Labour had won and had made the public believe that the Conservatives' NHS reforms were everything the public were against. The New Labour spin machine called the reforms privatisation by the back door, a two-tier NHS, and hospital bed cuts – everything the public did not want.

To some extent, this was our fault in the implementation of the policy. The fund holding scenario was perhaps the most patient-empowering reform ever: in the current waiting list situation, we would see the patients getting their operations done in the private hospital of their choice with their own bit of their NHS budget. That was all well and good, but the problem was that the Conservatives never got that across and so could never translate a winning formula into votes.

The fatal error in the scheme was that the then Conservative government expected the nurses and doctors to manage these changes without paying them more. I believe that if the nurses and doctors had been paid an extra amount as an incentive to be involved in fund holding or their trust management then we would not be in the mess we are today. But again, we failed to get our point across, or perhaps we didn't really realise our own point. The point was to allow everyone in the health service who worked at the front line to get real power over the way they provided their service to their patients. This in turn would create competition within the service and allow choice and better standards for the patient.

This new style of reform, and front line management, involved more work for the clinicians and real trust from the then government. Small was beautiful, from the GP practice to the NHS Trust. That was the internal market, where money for a patient's care followed the patient. This, the internal market, was what New Labour spun to be the destroyer of the NHS. I believe that there are many in today's NHS who did not really realise the opportunities that those reforms offered at the time, and now look back on that time as one of missed opportunity. The unions, and I include the BMA, never really understood the opportunity that they had. The government neither explained the opportunities to them nor recognise the need to pay more to the clinicians for the delivery of reform.

The Conservatives were perceived as being arrogant and dismissive of the health service, and that attitude contributed to the New Labour landslide victory.

That was the past, but here we are today – New Labour has had our NHS for five years now and has dismantled the 'internal market'. In its place we have a massive, centralised, bureaucratic and often incompetent management structure strangling the service.

We have seen the merging of trust hospitals into super-trusts, primary care trusts created, and GP practices linked up to larger primary care groups or local health care co-operatives. We seem to have more managers and administrators than ever, often with little or no NHS experience. We have a government 'committed' to sorting out the problems, but the problems just seem to be getting worse – whether it be waiting lists, teenage pregnancies or postcode medicine. For us at the front line, it feels as if we have a government in charge which is thrashing about trying to be all things to all people: one day promising the patients that they can have their operations abroad if they have to wait too long here, another that the post code lottery has stopped and another that the new inclusive management structures will bring real change.

It just feels like what it is: money going to keep people in offices doing the easy bit – making up rules, typing up reports, organising restructuring and social inclusion, overloading the front line with meaningless bureaucracy. The people at the front line are fed up; more and more patients are rightly getting frustrated with the service, and are going privately for their treatment.

This is real social exclusion. Health is a bit like education – most people pay their taxes to get a good health service and a good education service. They only go privately if the state service is not good enough – there will always be a few exceptions, but this is the normal state of things. If we want social inclusion we have to make sure that the service keeps the majority of people on board with it, and in a democracy the only way to do that is to make the NHS so good that everyone wants to use it.

At present the service is struggling: the government is spending its money on managers and gizmos such as NHS Direct, and the patient is suffering. The morale within the health service is at an all-time low, and if we are not careful we are going to end up with a health service which won't work for either the patients or the people who work in it. Then we really will end up with two tier health care those who can afford to will pay, and those who can't will be left in whatever system is left.

Make no mistake, the private sector will grow, and take with it the best staff. I am not against this happening – it is in the spirit of competition – but as a one-nation Conservative I believe firmly in social inclusion. Therefore I believe in the need for a National Health Service free at the point of need, with the needs of the patient, and excellence in teaching, training and research at its heart. The private sector can exist for those who want it, but I believe any reforms should be aimed at making the NHS so good that the private sector is not in much demand.

I also believe that we should be funding our NHS out of taxation as it is the fairest and most efficient way to do it. There is no point in having loads of expensive bureaucracy in place in order to collect the tax. It is not just about the money, though, and we have to remember that. That is why the Conservative health policy and ideology must be so carefully thought out. We have a microcosm in the UK – Scotland, whose health spending is 23 per cent higher than England's, already at the European average, has already over the past five years seen waiting lists lengthen, increases in teenage pregnancies, and an explosion in the use of the private sector. So it is easy to see that something is deeply wrong, something that cannot be solved just by pumping in funding.

So what are my dreams for our floundering party, and our beloved (don't forget how lucky we are to have it) NHS?

First, we have to establish ourselves as real believers in our NHS. At present we have no credibility. New Labour are losing theirs, but we are still not gaining any, and I think that we have to be big enough to recognise the perception that people have: that the Conservative party is somehow out to destroy the NHS. This I know is not true, but we have to change how we are perceived. If we don't to that then I really think that we will see New Labour in power for a very long time – they are already talking about hopes to stay in power for most of this century. We need to get more of our real beliefs out there.

Second, my dream is that the NHS workers see the Conservative Party as the empowering party – the party which wants to cut out all the red tape, layers of administration and silly rules, and really trust the professionals to run budgets and manage the service, with the managers helping rather than telling from high what needs to be done. In my dream, this new clinical and financial power would give the clinicians more control over their work, allow them to do it better, and make NHS employment more professionally rewarding. They could and should earn more for reaching agreed targets and set standards, and for running budgets. The patients would feel more empowered knowing that their clinicians had control of their bit of their budget, and they could choose where to go and therefore get better care. In my dream, all of us would feel privileged to be involved in the teaching and training of the next generation of NHS nurses and doctors, and it would be the accepted norm for all patients to understand and be proud of this as part of their contribution to our NHS.

Third, we need a new type of hospital, called a 'step down' hospital. These should be for the patients who no longer need acute beds, but just need recovery beds, or beds on the way to residential or nursing care. These 'step down' hospitals would be low tech, and perhaps community based, but they would mean that every bed in the acute sector would be available to be used appropriately.

Fourth, we need to be realistic about our new hospitals and build for the future. No longer do people want the city centre site with no parking. New hospitals should be built on the outskirts of towns with free transport links and parking provided.

Fifth, NHS workers should get a tax break – to make them feel in part owners of the service they provide.

Sixth, we need to build on the fundholding model, which used competition as its driving force for increasing clinical standards. Instead of competition being our mantra, perhaps we have to think of co-opetition – co-operation and competition together helping improve the service to the patient.

Seventh, we need to get the community care budget into the health budget. This would allow for seamless care of the elderly, without the tangle of social work red tape.

Eighth, we need to commit ourselves to national disease targets already set by New Labour.

Ninth, we need to allow the academic professionals the space, time and respect to do their research, and encourage links with the drug companies who provide much of the resources for research. We need the clinicians to embrace management, and therefore regain their professional power. We have to help them understand that the Conservatives are the party of trust.

Finally, I know that I am one of the lucky ones. I went to a comprehensive school, and then medical school where I didn't have to pay any fees. I worked my 100+ hours a week as a junior doctor and loved every minute of it. I never gave how much money I earned a thought as I enjoyed the job so much. I entered general practice in 1990, and saw things for patients start to get better. Now I am seeing them getting worse again. Worse still, I am seeing the morale in the health service dwindle to an all time low, and I am seeing the service start to collapse.

The answer is not just money. It is time to get the meddling politicians – who haven't got a clue what life at the front line is about – out of our NHS. It is time to depoliticise and reprofessionalise it.

Why can't the Conservatives champion that?

Appendix

The NHS In Crisis?

Stephen Evans and Sean Williams,

Policy Unit, the Conservative Party

Few debates contain more passionate or diverse voices than the health debate. Many of these voices are contained within this volume. They set out clear agendas for reform which those involved in public policy making should listen to. The Conservative party is listening. Inevitably, some of the contributions in this volume will be more influential than others on our approach.

This appendix attempts to set down the facts. People involved in the debate, and many of our activists, often ask us for an overview of some of the key factors that can be used to describe the state of the NHS. Inevitably, it is all too easy to produce one figure to prove a point, either in defence or attack of the system, and some might suggest that we have not set out all the relevant data. We will examine the data in terms of:

- Public Perceptions
- Waiting lists
- Waiting times

- Cancelled operations
- Levels of throughput
- Health outcomes
- Opt outs
- Regional differences within the UK

Public Perceptions

We set out below data from a recent Gallup poll:

	% of people agreeing
The Health Service is in	
• peak condition	1%
• reasonably good health	33%
• somewhat failing health	46%
• very poor condition	19%
Overall the NHS is	
• getting better	13%
• staying about the same	45%
• getting worse	40%
People believe that	
• waiting times for operations are often far too long	89%
• Accident and emergency waiting times are often far too long	83%
• There is a lot of bad management and waste in the NHS	82%

Source: Gallup 2002 for the *Daily Telegraph*

Waiting Lists

The NHS suffers from one of the largest healthcare waiting lists in the world. In the UK as a whole it stood at over 1.2 million people in September 2001. That is more than 10% of all annual inpatient admissions. It means that 2% of the whole population in the UK is waiting for hospital treatment at any one time.

The chart below shows the trend in waiting lists since March 1997. In March 1997, the waiting list for the UK stood at 1.36 million; in September 2001 it remained at 1.24 million. That is a reduction of less than 2% per year over the period. At the current rate of decrease, the UK waiting list would not be cleared until 2042.

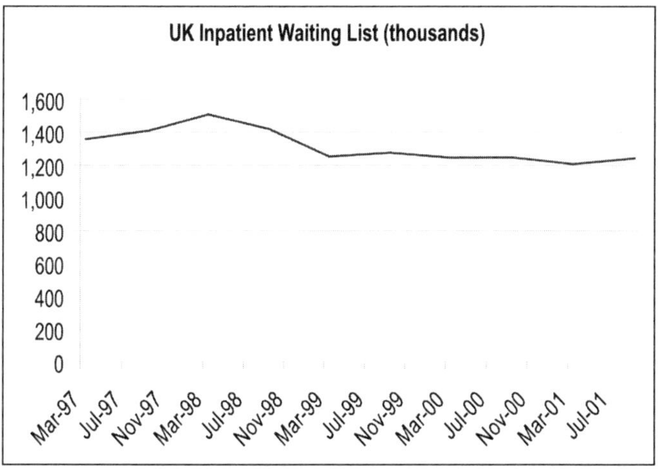

UK Inpatient Waiting List (thousands)

Source: Hospital Waiting Lists in England; NHS Wales: Hospital Waiting Lists; Waiting List Briefing, ISD Scotland; Northern Ireland Waiting Lists, DHSSPS Northern Ireland

Having waiting lists stuck at over a million people is clearly not a desirable outcome from the British health system.

Waiting Times

A target of six months maximum waiting time has been set, to be reached by 2005.

The percentage of patients waiting over 12 months has increased in 80% of all health authorities since 1997.

Percentage of patients on in-patient waiting list over 12 months

Health Authority	Mar-97	Aug-01	Increase
Bedfordshire	1.3%	7.0%	538%
Birmingham	0.1%	2.0%	2000%
Cornwall	0.8%	5.1%	638%
Dudley	0.2%	2.2%	1100%
East Kent	0.5%	6.9%	1380%
Gloucestershire	0.1%	1.6%	1600%
North Cheshire	0.9%	7.9%	878%
North Cumbria	0.1%	1.8%	1800%
Shropshire	0.2%	3.5%	1750%
Somerset	0.2%	3.4%	1700%
South & West Devon	0.1%	6.6%	6600%
South Staffordshire	0.2%	5.2%	2600%
Wigan & Bolton	0.6%	3.7%	617%

Source: Parl Deb, 1/11/01, 817 w

In addition, overall average waiting times for both inpatients and outpatients rose in all regions over the last quarter:

Average waiting time in days, England, all specialities

Period	Inpatients	Outpatients	Total
2001 Q1	130.7	67.1	197.8
2001 Q2	136	61.8	197.7
2001 Q3	136.5	64.3	200.8

Source: Health Care Navigator NHS Patient Waiting Times Monitor, edition 6

In some cases, the fight to clear waiting lists is actually self-defeating. Recent figures show that the number of patients who have to be readmitted as emergency cases after they had been discharged has increased significantly over the last year, by nearly 20% in some hospitals.

In addition, 5,000 patients a year die from diseases that they picked up whilst actually being treated in hospitals for other illnesses.

Waiting times of this nature are also clearly not a desirable outcome of the British health system. It has to be remembered that 14% of people waiting for treatment experience a high level of pain, and 40% experience at least some.

Cancelled operations

A related symptom of the way the NHS is managed is the number of operations that simply never happen. Cancelled operations now stand at around 80,000 per year.

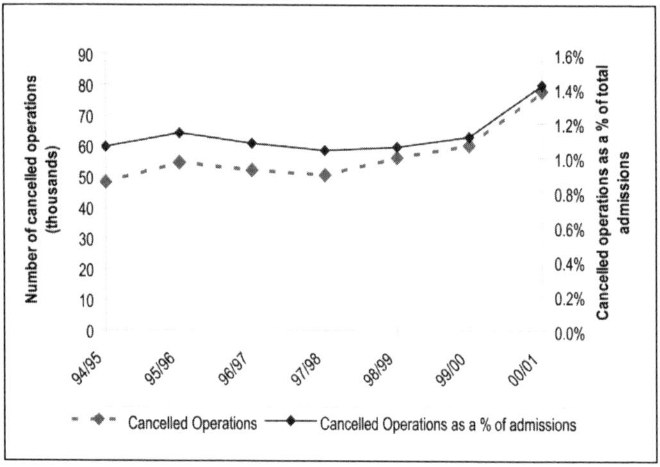

Source: Quarterly Statistics on Cancelled Operations; HC Deb 31/1/02, column 550-1 w

Levels of Throughput

Waiting lists, waiting times and cancelled operations are all measures of the capacity problems in the NHS. The principal measure of its capacity is the level of throughput in terms of admissions. Patient throughput is declining.

Hospital In-patient Admissions (England)

Year	Admissions	Year-on-year change
1990–91	8,188,087	
1991–92	8,724,328	6.5%
1992–93	9,078,863	4.1%
1993-94	9,492,652	4.6%
1994-95	9,857,320	3.8%
1995-96	10,247,000	4.0%
1996-97	10,190,689	-0.5%
1997-98	10,537,535	3.4%
1998-99	10,708,972	1.6%
1999-00	11,025,944	3.0%
2000-01	11,001,095	-0.2%

Source: Parl deb, 13/12/01 Column 982w

Health Outcomes

Perhaps the most powerful measure of the performance of the NHS is the health outcomes it delivers relative to other countries.

The NHS cannot be held solely responsible for the prevalence of diseases in the country. That depends on many factors, most of them outside the control of the NHS. However, the NHS can be measured for its performance in helping people recover once a disease has been contracted and treatment given. As such, survival rates – the proportion of people who survive for five years after treatment – is a good measure of how effective that treatment has been.

In terms of health outcomes, the UK compares unfavourably with much of Europe and America. An international comparison of survival rates of people suffering from various forms of cancer in the late 1980s, measuring how many people survive five years after their treatment, shows that people in Europe and America were much more likely to survive five years than people in England. For ovarian cancer, for example, survival rates are 20% better in Europe and 50% better in America. For prostate cancer, survival rates are 33% better in Europe and over 100% better in America.

Relative Cancer Survival Rates – Europe and America relative to the UK

Cancer Type	UK	Europe	America
Lung – Men	1.00	1.67	2.17
Lung – Women	1.00	1.83	2.67
Stomach – Men	1.00	2.10	1.80
Stomach – Women	1.00	2.18	2.27
Colon – Men	1.00	1.21	1.64
Colon – Women	1.00	1.21	1.62
Liver – Men	1.00	2.50	1.50
Liver – Women	1.00	2.50	4.00
Kidney – Men	1.00	1.23	1.48

cont'd

Cancer Type	UK	Europe	America
Kidney – Women	1.00	1.39	1.56
Breast (Women)	1.00	1.07	1.24
Ovary (Women)	1.00	1.21	1.55
Prostate (Men)	1.00	1.33	2.05
All leukaemias – Men	1.00	1.26	1.52
All leukaemias – Women	1.00	1.30	1.41

Source: ONS. Period 1986 – 90

Over a decade on, nothing has changed. Survival rates in England for many cancers remain frighteningly low:

Five-year survival of patients diagnosed in 1992-94, England (%)

	Male	Female
Oesophagus	6.7	7.7
Stomach	11.1	11.8
Colon	43.5	43.3
Lung	5.5	5.5
Breast	n/a	75.9
Cervix	66.0	n/a
Prostate	59.8	n/a
Bladder	67.1	57.6

Source: ONS

Opt Outs

Over a quarter of a million people are choosing to self-fund their operations in the private sector this year. Moreover, the number is growing- BUPA reported a 30% growth in self-pay patients between 1998 and 2000.

In addition, the take up of private medical insurance for those that can afford it has grown by 5% in the last year. According to one source (www.tradeunion-privatehealth.org.uk), 3.5 million out of 6.8 million TUC aligned trade unionists have some form of private health funding.

The Lessons from UK Countries

In all parts of the UK except England, spending is already well above the government's spending target of 8% of GDP.

Total Health Spending in UK Countries

Country	1999-2000% of GDP
England	7.3%
Wales	9.1%
Scotland	8.6%
Northern Ireland	9.2%

Source: NHS expenditure data from regional health authorities: DOH; Scottish Budget 2002/3; Welsh Assembly budget tables; Northern Ireland finance directorate

The table below shows the waiting lists in each of the countries of the UK, in absolute numbers and as a number of people on the waiting list out of each 1,000 people in the population. It can be seen that, although Northern Ireland and Wales have higher levels of spending than England, they also have higher waiting lists. In the case of Northern Ireland there are 50% more people on the waiting lists than there are in England.

Waiting Lists in the UK

	England	Wales	Scotland	NI	UK Total
Waiting Lists (000's) (30/09/01)	1,035.3	68.5	81.3	56.7	1,241.8
Population(000s)	49,494	2,934	5,120	1,689	59,237
Waiting Lists (Per 1,000 population)	20.9	23.3	15.9	33.6	21.0

Source: House of Commons Library

A similar picture emerges when health outcomes are considered. The table below shows the mortality rates for the four countries arising from heart disease, some forms of cancer and also for infants. It shows that higher spending does not necessarily result in better outcomes. On many measures, Scotland, Wales and Northern Ireland have worse outcomes than the UK and the EU as a whole, despite the higher levels of spending.

Health Outcomes for UK CountriesAge standardised mortality per 100,000 population 1998

Coronary heart disease, men and women under 75

Country	Male	Female
Scotland	207	80
Northern Ireland	188	67
England and Wales	159	56
EU	1510	633

Breast cancer for women aged under 75

Country	Female
Scotland	35
England and Wales	34
Northern Ireland	34
EU	1530

Lung cancer for men and women aged under 75

Country	Male	Female
Scotland	78	42
England and Wales	57	29
Northern Ireland	55	30
EU	156	715

Still births, perinatal and infant mortality per 1,000 births 1999

	Still Births	Perinatal mortality	Infant mortality
England	5.3	8.2	5.7
Wales	4.8	7.8	6.4
Scotland	5.2	7.6	5.0
Northern Ireland	5.7	10.0	6.4

Source: House of Commons Library

In Scotland, a third more people die of heart disease and 40% more people die of lung disease than in England. It is also true that fewer people survive for five years after their treatment for heart disease or lung disease in Scotland than they do in England.

The picture is the same in Wales and Northern Ireland. They spend a lot more on health than England, but they actually have more people on their waiting lists than England, relative to the size of their populations. In fact, we spend more on health in Northern Ireland than they do in the Republic of Ireland, but we have more people on waiting lists (relative to population) and worse healthcare.

Conclusion

The facts speak for themselves. The NHS as currently run is not delivering the level of service that patients in Britain deserve. It is a system in chronic need of reform. It is against the background of these facts that the Conservative Party is developing policies to improve the healthcare which people in Britain enjoy.